Drug Update

A Compendium

Drug Update
A Compendium

Maheshi Chhaya MBBS MD (Pharmacology)

Tutor
Department of Pharmacology
HBT Medical College and
Dr RN Cooper Municipal General Hospital
Mumbai

Disha Rambhia MBBS MD (Pharmacology) DBM

Tutor
Department of Pharmacology
HBT Medical College and
Dr RN Cooper Municipal General Hospital
Mumbai

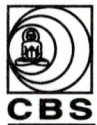

CBS

CBS Publishers and Distributors Pvt Ltd

New Delhi • Bengaluru • Chennai • Kochi • Kolkata • Mumbai
Bhopal • Bhubaneswar • Hyderabad • Jharkhand • Nagpur • Patna
Pune • Uttarakhand • Dhaka (Bangladesh) • Kathmandu (Nepal)

Drug Update
A Compendium

ISBN: 978-81-94125-49-5

Copyright © Authors and Publisher

First Edition: 2019

Published by Satish Kumar Jain and produced by Varun Jain for

CBS Publishers and Distributors Pvt Ltd

4819/XI Prahlad Street, 24 Ansari Road, Daryaganj, New Delhi 110 002, India.

Ph: 23289259, 23266861, 23266867   Website: www.cbspd.com

Fax: 011-23243014   e-mail: delhi@cbspd.com; cbspubs@airtelmail.in.

Corporate Office: 204 FIE, Industrial Area, Patparganj, Delhi 110 092

Ph: 4934 4934   Fax: 4934 4935   e-mail: publishing@cbspd.com;
publicity@cbspd.com

Branches

- **Bengaluru:** Seema House 2975, 17th Cross, K.R. Road, Banasankari 2nd Stage, Bengaluru 560 070, Karnataka
  Ph: +91-80-26771678/79   Fax: +91-80-26771680   e-mail: bangalore@cbspd.com
- **Chennai:** 7, Subbaraya Street, Shenoy Nagar, Chennai 600 030, Tamil Nadu
  Ph: +91-44-26680620, 26681266   Fax: +91-44-42032115   e-mail: chennai@cbspd.com
- **Kochi:** 68/1534, 35, 36 Power House Road, Opp. KSEB, Kochi 682018, Kerala
  Ph: +91-484-4059061-65   Fax: +91-484-4059065   e-mail: kochi@cbspd.com
- **Kolkata:** 6/B, Ground Floor, Rameswar Shaw Road, Kolkata-700 014, West Bengal
  Ph: +91-33-22891126, 22891127, 22891128 e-mail: kolkata@cbspd.com
- **Mumbai:** 83-C, Dr E Moses Road, Worli, Mumbai-400018, Maharashtra
  Ph: +91-22-24902340/41   Fax: +91-22-24902342   e-mail: mumbai@cbspd.com

Representatives

Bhopal	0-8319310552	Bhubaneswar	0-9911037372	Hyderabad	0-9885175004
Jharkhand	0-9811541605	Nagpur	0-9421945513	Patna	0-9334159340
Pune	0-9623451994	Uttarakhand	0-9716462459	Dhaka	01912-003485
Kathmandu (Nepal)	977-9818742655			(Bangladesh)	

Printed at India Binding House, Noida, UP, India

Foreword

I have been acquainted with the dedication of Dr Maheshi Chhaya and Dr Disha Rambhia towards their work since they were postgraduate residents in the department of pharmacology. I, as the Head of Department of Pharmacology at HBT Medical College and Dr RN Cooper Municipal General Hospital, 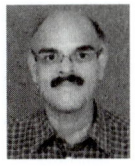 Mumbai, am poised with the proficiency and sincerity of Dr Maheshi and Dr Disha in their capacity as educators.

Innovations in technology have accelerated the course of drug discovery. With each medical breakthrough, the horizon for providing a rational treatment widens, impinging on the already far reaching ethical dilemmas surrounding patient care. Thus, necessitating a 'know-all' for those practicing medicine.

Drug Update—A Compendium captures the enthusiastic perseverance of Dr Maheshi Chhaya and Dr Disha Rambhia towards taking forward the mantle of continued medical education. They have transcribed the overwhelming information surrounding new drug approvals and drug safety updates into a simple, comprehensive and lucid design that will aid medical education and clinical decision making.

Dr Prasad Pandit
Professor and Head
Department of Pharmacology
HBT Medical College and
Dr RN Cooper Municipal General Hospital
Mumbai

Preface

We belong to an era where each day unfolds new corners in our understanding of the medical science and every new piece of evidence enables us to make clinically pertinent and rational decisions towards our patients. With 'Drug Update—A Compendium', we intend to provide a platform that will gratify the gap between the expeditious pace of medical development and its clinical awareness. Here we provide a carefully curated manuscript that talks about advancements in medical pharmacology, the landscape of which covers global new drug approvals and safety updates. Each chapter reviews the new drug within the scope of its clinical pharmacology and therapeutic implications. Major feature of our book is the portrayal of each molecule in the light of already available data and the quick review index at the start of each chapter.

What started off as a small project of exchanging drug update summaries between colleagues, became the very pillar of foundation for this book as well as the deep-rooted friendship that we share with each other today. The journey from colleagues to co-authors made us grow not only as individuals but also as clinicians and academicians.

We would like to thank "Ramesh Krishnamachari" of CBS Publishers and Distributors for providing the correct direction to our journey. Suggestions and comments towards the betterment of 'Drug Update—A Compendium' would be most welcome. They may be sent to us in the care of the publishers.

Maheshi Chhaya
Disha Rambhia

Acknowledgements

At the outset, we would like to take this opportunity to articulate our gratitude to our respected and learned mentors at the Department of Pharmacology, Topiwala National Medical College and BYL Nair Ch. Hospital, Mumbai, for imparting us with the knowledge that helped us build the naissance of this project.

The fruitful accomplishment of this endeavor is attributable to the extraordinary guidance, the unremitting support and the profound motivation we received from the respected faculty at the Department of Pharmacology, Hinduhridaysamrat Balasaheb Thackeray Medical College and Dr RN Cooper Municipal General Hospital, Mumbai.

We are grateful to our family, friends and colleagues for their immense faith and the moral, emotional and physical support needed during the effective inscription of the book.

We thank the websites of US-FDA, Medscape, PubMed and DRUGBANK for their scientifically accurate, reliable and easily accessible data which helped shape our book.

Maheshi Chhaya
Disha Rambhia

Contents

1 | Drugs Acting on the Central Nervous System

	Drug	Class	Indication
1	Lofexidine	α receptor agonist	Opioid withdrawal
2	Erenumab-aooe	CGRP receptor antagonist	Migraine prophylaxis
3	Fremanezumab-vfrm	CGRP antagonist	Migraine prophylaxis
4	Galcanezumab-gnlm	CGRP antagonist	Migraine prophylaxis
5	Cannabidiol	Anticonvulsant	Lennox-Gastaut syndrome; Dravet syndrome
6	Stiripentol	Anticonvulsant	Dravet syndrome
7	Patisiran	Anti-transthyretin	Amyloidosis
8	Inotersen	Anti-transthyretin	Amyloidosis

Lofexidine α_2 Receptor Agonist

Approval—May 16, 2018

Indication

To mitigate opioid withdrawal symptoms so as to facilitate abrupt opioid discontinuation, in adults.

Mechanism of Action

Lofexidine is a centrally acting $\alpha2$ adrenergic receptor agonist. On binding to the $\alpha2$ receptors on the adrenergic neurons, lofexidine reduces the release of norepinephrine from them. This in turn reduces the sympathetic tone.

Pharmacokinetics

- Peaks at 3–5 hours, accumulates
- Follows first order kinetics
- Absolute bioavailability is 72%
- aVd (apparant volume of distribution) is 480L
- 55% plasma protein bound
- Metabolized by CYP2D6, majorly
- t½ is 12 hours, 17 to 22 hours at steady state

Adverse Drug Reactions, Warnings and Precautions

- The common ADRs are orthostatic hypotension, bradycardia, dizziness, somnolence, dry mouth; risk of QTc prolongation is present.
- Opioid overdose after opioid discontinuation is a possibility.
- Abrupt discontinuation may result in withdrawal symptoms.

Contraindications

None

Drug Interactions

- Increased risk of QTc prolongation with methadone.

3

- Reduced efficacy of naltrexone on concomitant administration.
- Increased CNS depression with CNS depressants.
- Increased plasma concentration with CYP2D6 inhibitors like paroxetine.

Posology

- Three 0.18 mg tablets to be taken orally 4 times a day at 5–6 hourly intervals for up to 14 days.
- Discontinuation to be gradual over 2–4 days.
- Doses to be reduced in patients with hepatic and renal impairment.
- Hepatic impairment: 3, 2, 1 tablet 4 times a day for mild, moderate, severe impairment, respectively.
- Renal impairment: 2, 1 tablet 4 times a day for mild to moderate and severe impairment, respectively.

Limitations

- Risk of cardiac rhythm abnormalities and/or QTc prolongation exists when used in individuals with cardiac rhythm abnormalities or drugs causing QTc prolongation.
- Caution to be exercised in those with hepatic and renal impairment.

Erenumab-aooe

CGRP Receptor Antagonist

Approval—May 17, 2018

Indication

Prophylaxis of migraine, in adults

Mechanism of Action

- Erenumab-aooe is a human IgG2 (monoclonal antibody) with high affinity for CGRP (calcitonin-gene related peptide) receptor.
- CGRP binds with the CGRP receptor and modulates nociceptive signaling and is said to promote migraine.
- Erenumab-aooe prevents the binding of CGRP with its receptors and thus prevents migraine.

Pharmacokinetics

- Peaks at 6 days
- Follows non-linear kinetics
- Steady state at 3 months
- Absolute bioavailability is 82%.
- t½ is 28 days.
- Elimination is biphasic—at low concentration, binding to receptors; at high concentration, nonspecific proteolysis.

Adverse Drug Reactions, Warnings and Precautions

- The common ADRs are injection site reactions, constipation, muscle spasms.
- Cautious use in pregnancy is recommended as it is found to be safe according to animal data but human studies are lacking.
- Not tried in patients with severe hepatic or renal impairment.

Contraindications

None

Drug Interactions

None

Posology

- 70 or 140 mg once a month
- 140 mg to be administered as two consecutive injections of 70 mg
- *Route:* Subcutaneous
- *Site:* Abdomen, thigh, upper arm

Advantages

- Does not interact with the drugs used for migraine treatment.
- Once a month dosing enhances compliance.
- Can be self-administered.

Limitations

- Cannot be used to treat an acute attack of migraine.

Fremanezumab-vfrm   CGRP antagonist

Approval—September 14, 2018

Indication

Prophylaxis of migraine, in adults

Mechanism of Action

- Fremanezumab-vfrm is a humanized IgG2Aa/kappa monoclonal antibody against the CGRP ligand.
- By binding to CGRP, it prevents binding of CGRP to its receptor, thereby preventing downstream nociceptive signaling.

Pharmacokinetics

- Peaks at 5 to 7 days
- Steady state at 6 months
- aVd is 6 L
- Metabolized by proteolysis
- t½ is 31 days.

Adverse Drug Reactions, Warnings and Precautions

- Injection site reactions are the most common ADRs.
- Hypersensitivity reactions like rash, pruritus, urticaria may occur.

Contraindications

Hypersensitivity to Fremanezumab-vfrm or any excipients

Drug Interactions

None

Posology

- 225 mg once a month
  OR
- 675 mg every 3 months as 3 consecutive injections of 225 mg

Route: Subcutaneous
Site: Abdomen, thigh, upper arm

7

Advantages

⊕ No dose adjustments required pertaining to age, gender, race or weight.

⊕ Can be self-administered.

Limitations

⊕ No studies are performed in special population.

⊕ Safety in hepatic or renal impairment is not known.

⊕ Cannot be used for the treatment of migraine.

Galcanezumab-gnlm

CGRP Antagonist

Approval—September 27, 2018

Indication

Prophylaxis of migraine, in adults

Mechanism of Action

- Galcanezumab-gnlm is a humanized IgG4 monoclonal antibody directed against the CGRP ligand.
- It binds to CGRP, prevents its binding to CGRP receptor thereby preventing downstream nociceptive signaling.

Pharmacokinetics

- Peaks at 5 days
- aVd is 7.3 L
- Metabolized by proteolysis
- t½ is 27 days.

Adverse Drug Reactions, Warnings and Precautions

- Injection site reactions like pain, erythema, pruritus are the most common ADRs observed.
- Hypersensitivity reactions like rash, urticaria, dyspnea may occur. If the reaction is serious, stop the drug. Reactions may occur even after a few days of drug administration.

Contraindications

Hypersensitivity to Galcanezumab-gnlm or its excipients

Drug Interactions

None

Posology

Loading: 240 mg (as two consecutive injections of 120 mg)
Maintenance: 120 mg monthly

Route: Subcutaneous

Sites: Abdomen, thigh, back of the upper arm, buttocks

No studies in patients with hepatic or renal impairment. Dose reduction is, however, not needed in patients with mild to moderate renal impairment.

Advantages

- Pharmacokinetics not affected by age, sex, race or subtypes of migraine (episodic or chronic).
- Can be self-administered.

Limitations

- Delayed hypersensitivity reactions may occur; constant vigilance is needed.
- Data on special population is lacking.
- Cannot be used for the treatment of migraine.

Cannabidiol   Anticonvulsant

Approval—June 25, 2018

Indication

Treatment of seizures associated with Lennox-Gastaut syndrome and Dravet syndrome, in those aged 2 years or more

Mechanism of Action

Majorly unknown, some postulations are

- Antagonism of CB1 and CB2, *in vitro*, responsible for the lack of psychotropic effects
- Activation of $5-HT_{1A}$ receptors
- Reduction of the synaptic release of glutamate antagonizing G protein-coupled receptor (GPR) 55
- Stimulation and desensitization of transient receptor potential of vanilloid type 1 (TRPV1) and 2 (TRPV2) channels
- Inhibition of the synaptic uptake of GABA, noradrenaline, adenosine, dopamine
- Stimulation of 3 and 1 glycine receptors
- Stimulation and desensitization of transient receptor potential of ankyrin type 1 (TRPA1) channel
- Other targets are COX, NO, PPAR-gamma, GPR18, voltage-dependent anion channel 1 (VDAC1), TNF, fatty acid amide hydrolase (FAAH)

Pharmacokinetics

- Peaks at 2.5 to 5 hours
- aVd is 20963 to 42849 L
- t½ is 56 to 61 hours
- Metabolized, in liver and gut, by CYP2C19, CYP3A4 enzymes, and UGT1A7, UGT1A9, UGT2B7 isoforms
- Excreted in feces with minor renal clearance

Adverse Drug Reactions, Warnings and Precautions

- Common ADRs include somnolence, anorexia, diarrhea, fatigue, malaise, asthenia, rash, insomnia, infections, transaminase elevations.
- Monitoring of serum transaminases before and after initiation is necessary as hepatocellular injury may occur.
- Risk of somnolence/sedation is more if used with CNS depressants. Individuals must refrain from driving or operating heavy machinery.
- Monitoring for suicidal behavior and ideation is a must.
- In case of a hypersensitivity reaction, the drug needs to be discontinued.
- Cannabidiol should be withdrawn gradually in order to prevent precipitation of status epilepticus.

Contraindications

- Hypersensitivity to Cannabidiol or its excipients
- Pregnancy: May cause fetal harm

Drug Interactions

- Reduce dose if used with a CYP3A4 or CYP2C19 inhibitor, increase dose if used with an inducer.
- Reduce dose of concomitantly used substrates of UGT1A9, UGT2B7, CYP2C8, CYP2C9, CYP2C19
- Start at a lower dose in elderly.

Posology

- 2.5 mg/kg orally twice daily
- After a week, dose can be increased to 5 mg/kg twice daily (maximum recommended maintenance dose is 10 mg/kg twice daily)
- Dose reduction is needed in those with moderate to severe hepatic impairment.

Advantages

- Efficacious in refractory seizures
- No abuse or dependence causing potential
- No withdrawal symptoms on discontinuation.

Limitations

- Can cause hepatic injury.

Stiripentol | Anticonvulsant

Approval—August 20, 2018

Indication

Treatment of seizures associated with Dravet syndrome in patients aged 2 years and above, as add-on therapy

Mechanism of Action

Unknown, possible mechanisms include:
- Direct effects mediated through $GABA_A$ receptors
- Indirect effects involving inhibition of cytochrome P450 activity resulting in an increase in the plasma concentration of its substrates like clobazam

Pharmacokinetics

- Peaks at 2 to 3 hours
- Plasma protein binding is 99%.
- Metabolized by CYP1A2, CYP2C19, CYP3A4 in the liver
- $t\frac{1}{2}$ is 4.5 to 13 hours but increases in a dose-dependent manner.

Adverse Drug Reactions, Warnings and Precautions

- Common ADRs are somnolence, anorexia, weight loss, hypotonia, nausea, tremor, dysarthria, insomnia.
- Neutropenia and thrombocytopenia may occur. Monitoring is essential.
- Withdrawal of the drug should be gradual.
- Suicidal thoughts and behavior may occur.
- Since the drug contains phenylalanine, cautious approach is needed in patient with phenylketonuria.

Contraindications

Pregnancy: May cause fetal harm

Drug Interactions

- An inhibitor of CYP3A4, CYP2C19, CYP2C8, CYP1A2, CYP2B6, P-gp, BCRP. Substrates need dose reduction.
- Increase in its plasma concentration may be seen when co-administered with drugs inhibiting cytochrome P450 enzymes.

Posology

50 mg/kg/day in 2–3 divided doses, orally, during a meal.

Capsule: As a whole with a glass of water

Suspension: Mixed in a glass of water and taken immediately

Advantages

- Effective in refractory seizures.

Limitations

- Efficacy and safety in special population is not known.

Patisiran   Anti-Transthyretin

Approval—August 10, 2018

Indication

Treatment of hereditary transthyretin-mediated amyloidosis (hATTR) induced polyneuropathy, in adults

Mechanism of Action

- Patisiran is a small interfering ribonucleic acid (siRNA), formulated as a lipid complex so as to reach the hepatocytes.
- Within the hepatocytes, it brings about the degradation of the mutant and wild-type TTR (transthyretin) mRNA through RNA interference resulting in the reduction in serum TTR proteins and thus TTR protein deposits in the tissues.

Pharmacokinetics

- Steady state at 24 weeks
- Low plasma protein binding, ≤2.1%
- Distributes to the liver
- Metabolized by nucleases
- <1% is excreted unchanged in urine
- t½ ranges from 3.2 ±1.8 days

Adverse Drug Reactions, Warnings and Precautions

- Common ADRs are URTIs, infusion reactions, dyspepsia, dyspnea, muscle spasms, arthralgia, erythema, bronchitis, vertigo.
- To prevent infusion-related reactions, pretreat with corticosteroid, acetaminophen and antihistamines (H1 and H2 blockers). If the reaction is serious or life-threatening, the drug has to be stopped.
- Reduction of serum vitamin A levels is observed. Supplementation is recommended. In case of visual abnormalities, an ophthalmologist should be consulted.

Contraindications

None

Drug Interactions

None

Posology

Varies according to body weight:
- <100 kg—0.3 mg/kg once every 3 weeks
- >100 kg—30 mg once every 3 weeks

Administered as an IV infusion over 80 minutes. Filter and dilute prior to administration.

Advantages

- Patisiran is the first drug of its kind.
- No dose alteration is required in the elderly or those with mild to moderate renal or hepatic impairment.

Limitations

- Efficacy and safety in pregnant, lactating women and children is not known.

Inotersen

Anti-Transthyretin

Approval—October 5, 2018

Indication

Treatment of amyloidogenic transthyretin amyloidosis-associated polyneuropathy, in adults

Mechanism of Action

- Inotersen is an antisense oligonucleotide against the TTR protein.
- By binding to the TTR mRNA, it causes degradation of mutant and wild-type TTR mRNA.
- This results in a reduction of serum TTR protein and thus TTR protein deposits in tissues.

Pharmacokinetics

- Peaks at 2 to 4 hours
- >94% bound to plasma proteins
- High concentration in liver, kidney
- Does not cross the blood–brain barrier
- aVd is 293L
- Metabolized by nucleases
- <1% is excreted unchanged in urine
- t½ is 32.3 days

Adverse Drug Reactions, Warnings and Precautions

- Common ADRs include injection site reactions, nausea, headache, fever, fatigue, thrombocytopenia.
- Stroke or cervicocephalic arterial dissection may occur within 2 days of onset of treatment along with symptoms of cytokine release.
- Inflammatory and immune effects may present as serious neurological side effects.
- Monitoring liver enzymes every 4 months during therapy is required as they may rise during treatment.
- Hypersensitivity reactions and reduction in serum vitamin A level may occur (supplementation is recommended).
- May cause QTc prolongation.

Black Box Warning

⊕ Sudden and unpredictable, potentially life-threatening, thrombocytopenia can occur, monitoring is advised.
⊕ Glomerulonephritis requiring immunosuppressive therapy, potentially leading to dialysis dependent renal failure, is a possibility. Monitoring for the same before and after onset of treatment is required.

Contraindications

⊕ Platelet count <100 x 10^9/L
⊕ History of acute glomerulonephritis with Inotersen
⊕ History of hypersensitivity to Inotersen

Drug Interactions

⊕ Caution is advised when co-administered with anticoagulants, anti-platelet and nephrotoxic drugs.
⊕ Not a substrate/inducer/inhibitor of CYP450 enzymes.

Posology

⊕ 284 mg subcutaneously, once a week.
⊕ Laboratory tests, before, during and 8 weeks after discontinuation of treatment are essential.

Advantages

⊕ The first of its kind.

Limitations

⊕ Cannot be administered in patients with low platelet counts, hepatic/renal disease/impairment.
⊕ Additional adverse effects like CHF, chills, myalgia, extremity pain may be seen in the elderly.
⊕ Efficacy and safety in the pregnant, lactating women and children is not known.

2
Drugs Acting on the Respiratory System

	Drug	Class	Indication
1	Tezacaftor/ Ivacaftor	CFTR modulator	Cystic fibrosis
2	Revefenacin	Long-acting muscarinic agonist	Chronic obstructive pulmonary disease

Tezacaftor/Ivacaftor   CFTR Modulator

Approval—February 12, 2018

Indication

Treatment of cystic fibrosis in patients with homozygous *F508del* mutation or at least one mutation in the CFTR (cystic fibrosis transmembrane conductance regulator) gene responsive to tezacaftor/ivacaftor, in those aged >12 years

Mechanism of Action

- The *F508del* mutation causes a processing and trafficking defect that causes reduction in the amount of protein on the epithelial membrane. It also interrupts the gating of the few channels that reach the surface. All this results in minimal CFTR-mediated chloride transport.
- Tezacaftor is a new molecule which acts as a CFTR corrector, it modifies the cellular processing and trafficking of the CFTR protein thereby, increasing the amount of normally functioning CFTR at the cell surface.
- On the other hand, Ivacaftor, which is a CFTR potentiator, increases the channel gating activity of protein kinase A-activated CFTR and enhancing the ion transport at the cell surface.
- Ivacaftor thus helps potentiate the CFTR protein delivered to the cell surface by Tezacaftor, further enhancing the chloride ion transport, more than that caused by either drug alone.

Pharmacokinetics

- Ivacaftor exposure increases 3 times when consumed with fatty food
- Both drugs have high plasma protein binding capacity (99%).
- aVd of Tezacaftor is 271 L while that of Ivacaftor is 207 L.
- Both are metabolized extensively by CYP3A4, 3A5.
- t½ for Tezacaftor—15 hours and for Ivacaftor—13 hours.
- Both are excreted in feces (majorly), urine (minor).

Adverse Drug Reactions, Warnings and Precautions

⊕ Common ADRs noted are headache, nausea, congestion of the sinuses, dizziness, serum transaminase elevation, cataract.

Drug Interactions

⊕ Reduce dose when co-administered with moderate or strong CYP3A inhibitors, toxicity can occur.

⊕ Levels of both drugs are decreased when they are coadministered with strong CYP3A inducers.

⊕ Ivacaftor is a weak P-gp inhibitor, levels of substrates of P-gp (e.g. digoxin, cyclosporine) may increase when co-administered.

Posology

⊕ Tezacaftor—100 mg, Ivacaftor—150 mg BD with fat-containing food.

⊕ Reduce dose in moderate to severe hepatic failure.

⊕ To be used cautiously in severe renal impairment.

Advantages

⊕ Unlike the earlier CFTR corrector Lumacaftor, Tezacaftor does not induce CYP3A4 enzymes and does not interfere with metabolism of Ivacaftor or any other drug used in cystic fibrosis.

⊕ Acceptable safety profile, reduces sweat chloride, improves pulmonary function.

Revefenacin   Anticholinergic (LAMA)

Approval—November 9, 2018

Indication

Maintenance treatment of chronic obstructive pulmonary disease (COPD)

Mechanism of Action

- Competitive, reversible, long-acting muscarinic antagonist (LAMA).
- Revefenacin has a similar affinity for all muscarinic receptor subtypes, i.e. M1–M5.
- Inhibition of M3 receptor in the bronchial smooth muscle causes bronchodilation and relieves the symptoms of COPD.

Pharmacokinetics

- Metabolized via hydrolysis to a major active metabolite
- Excreted via feces
- t½ ranges from 22–70 hours

Adverse Drug Reactions, Warnings and Precautions

- Common ADRs seen are cough, nasopharyngitis, URTI, headache and backache.
- Revefenacin should not to be used to treat acute symptoms or in those having an acute deterioration of COPD.
- Paradoxical bronchospasm, worsening of narrow-angle glaucoma and urinary retention and immediate hypersensitivity reactions may occur.

Contraindications

Hypersensitivity to the drugs or any of its component.

Drug Interactions

- Additive action seen when concomitantly used with other anticholinergic medications.

- Co-administration with OATP1B1 and OATP1B3 inhibitors (e.g. rifampicin, cyclosporine) may lead to an increase in exposure of the active metabolite.

Posology

- One 175 μg vial (3 mL) once daily.
- Inhalation with a standard jet nebulizer with a mouthpiece connected to an air compressor.

Advantages

- It is a novel, long-acting drug with a selective action and hence has a lesser propensity to cause systemic anticholinergic side effects.
- Compliance is better as the drug needs to be taken once daily.

3   Drugs Acting on the Cardiovascular System

	Drug	Class	Indication
1	Lanadelumab - flyo	Kallikrein inhibitor	Hereditary angioedema
2	Antihemophilic factor pegylated - aucl	Coagulation factor	Hemophilia A
3	Andexanet-alfa	Coagulation factor	Bleeding due to rivaroxaban or apixaban
4	Avatrombopag	Thrombopoietin receptor agonist	Thrombocytopenia
5	Lusutrombopag	Thrombopoietin receptor agonist	Thrombocytopenia
6	Fostamatinib di-sodium dehydrate	Syk Tyrosine kinase inhibitor	Thrombocytopenia

Lanadelumab-flyo   Kallikrein Inhibitor

Approval—August 23, 2018

Indication

Prophylaxis of hereditary angioedema (HAE) in patients aged 12 years or more

Mechanism of Action

- In HAE due to C1-inhibitor (C1-INH) deficiency or dysfunction, there is an uncontrolled increase in the plasma kallikrein activity owing to its dysregulation.
- Plasma kallikrein is a protease that cleaves high-molecular weight kininogen (HMWK) to generate cleaved HMWK (cHMWK) and bradykinin.
- Bradykinin is a potent vasodilator, increases the vascular permeability and causes the swelling and pain seen in HAE.
- Lanadelumab-flyo is a fully human monoclonal antibody (IgG1/ κ chain) that binds plasma kallikrein and inhibits its proteolytic activity, thus controlling the excess bradykinin generation in HAE patients.

Pharmacokinetics

- t½ is 2 weeks.

Adverse Drug Reactions, Warnings and Precautions

- Injection site reactions, upper respiratory infections, headache, rash, myalgia, dizziness, and diarrhea are the common ADRs.
- The drug is immunogenic.
- Hypersensitivity reactions may occur.

Contraindications

None

Drug Interactions

Drug interaction studies have not been conducted.

Posology

300 mg subcutaneously, every 2 weeks.

Advantages

- Previously approved prophylactic therapies include attenuated androgens (e.g. danazol) and a plasma derived C1 inhibitor (Cinryze, Shire).
- Androgens need to be taken on a daily basis and according to various studies, discontinuation due to side effects is seen in 25% of patients.
- The C1 inhibitor needs to be administered intravenously after every 3–4 days. Such repetitive injections can increase the risk of exposure to infections and loss of venous access.
- In the light of the above information lanadelumab-flyo, a monoclonal antibody becomes a novel promising approach towards prevention of HAE.

Antihemophilic Factor PEGylated-aucl

Coagulation Factor

Approval—August 30, 2018

Indication

Hemophilia A in patients aged >12 years requiring on-demand treatment as well as to control bleeding episodes, manage perioperative bleeding and as a prophylactic agent to reduce the frequency of bleeding episodes

Mechanism of Action

- Antihemophilic factor (recombinant) PEGylated-aucl is a site-specific recombinant DNA-derived, factor VIII concentrate.
- It replaces the missing coagulation factor VIII, however, only temporarily.
- The site-specific PEGylation in the A3 domain helps by reducing its binding to the physiological factor VIII clearance receptors, thereby, extending the half-life and providing a better bioavailability.

Pharmacokinetics

- t½ is 18–20 hours.

Adverse Drug Reactions, Warnings and Precautions

- Common ADRs experienced are headache, cough, nausea and fever.
- Hypersensitivity reactions may occur.
- Factor VIII neutralizing antibodies may be seen.
- Immune response to PEG patients (majorly seen in patients <6 years of age) primarily presents as either acute hypersensitivity reactions or loss of efficacy. Thus it is recommended to evaluate patients experiencing the above symptoms in the absence of detectable Factor VIII inhibitors, for possible bleeding or reduced recovery.

Contraindications

Hypersensitivity to the drug or its components (PEG, mouse or hamster proteins)

Posology

To control bleeding episodes and for perioperative management:
- Expected recovery: 1 IU/kg will increase the factor VIII level by 2 IU/dL.
- Required dose (IU): Body weight (kg) x desired factor VIII rise (% of normal or IU/dL) x reciprocal of expected recovery (or observed recovery, if available).
- Estimated increment of factor VIII (IU/dL or % of normal) = [Total Dose (IU)/body weight (kg)] x 2 (IU/dL per IU/kg).

As routine prophylaxis:
- 30–40 IU/kg twice weekly.

Route: Intravenous

Advantages

- Improved lifetime of factor VIII; less dosing frequency.

Limitations

Not for use:
- In children aged <12 years, owing to increased risk of hypersensitivity reactions.
- Previously untreated patients.
- Treatment of von Willebrand disease.

Andexanet-alfa   Coagulation Factor

Approval—May 3, 2018

Indication

Reverse the anticoagulation due to rivaroxaban or apixaban in cases of life-threatening or uncontrolled bleeding

Mechanism of Action

- Andexanet-alfa is a recombinant human factor Xa which is catalytically inactive but retains the structural activity, similar to that of endogenous factor Xa.
- Andexanet-alfa binds to and sequesters the factor Xa inhibitors, rivaroxaban and apixaban.
- Also, it binds to and inhibits the activity of tissue factor pathway inhibitor (TFPI) which is responsible for increasing tissue factor-initiated thrombin generation.

Pharmacokinetics

- t½ is 5–7 hours.

Adverse Drug Reactions, Warnings and Precautions

- UTIs and pneumonia are common.
- Thromboembolic events both arterial and venous, ischemic and cardiac events including sudden death have been reported.
- After treatment with andexanet-alfa, anticoagulant therapy should be reinitiated as and when medically appropriate.
- Re-elevation of anticoagulant levels or incomplete reversal of anticoagulant activity can occur.
- Immunogenic potential is present.

Posology

- Dose of andexanet-alfa depends on the factor Xa inhibitor administered, its dose and the time since its last dose.
- Administered as an IV bolus, 400/800 mg at a rate of 30 mg/min, followed by infusion of 4/8 mg/min for 2 hours.

31

Advantages

⊕ Despite having a better bleeding risk profile compared to vitamin K antagonists, there was the disadvantage of the risk of bleeding in the absence of an antidote with apixaban and rivaroxaban, which can now be addressed with the approval of Andexanet-alfa (first in class).

Limitations

⊕ The drug has received an accelerated approval based on its capacity to modify the baseline anti-factor Xa activity in healthy volunteers, its action on improving hemostasis has not yet been proven.

⊕ It is not effective for the treatment of bleeding related to factor Xa inhibitors other than apixaban and rivaroxaban and should not be used for the same.

⊕ The safety and efficacy of more than one dose is questionable as it has not been evaluated.

Avatrombopag

Thrombopoietic Receptor Agonist

Approval—May 21, 2018

Indication

Treatment of thrombocytopenia in adult patients of chronic liver disease scheduled to undergo a procedure

Mechanism of Action

- Avatrombopag is a second generation thrombopoietin receptor agonist (TPO-RA). It stimulates the proliferation and differentiation of megakaryocytes from the bone marrow progenitor cells and thus leads to an increase in the platelet production.
- It does not compete with thrombopoietin (TPO) for binding to its receptor but shows an additive action with TPO on platelet production.

Pharmacokinetics

- Food reduces absorption by 40–60%
- Metabolized by CYP2C9 and 3A4
- Excreted primarily in feces
- t½ is 19 hours.

Adverse Drug Reactions, Warnings and Precautions

- Common ADRs experienced are fever, pain in abdomen, nausea, headache, fatigue, peripheral edema and hyponatremia.
- Patients with chronic liver disease may experience thrombo-embolic complications, the risk is high in those with genetic prothrombotic conditions like factor V Leiden, prothrombin 20210A, antithrombin deficiency, or protein C or S deficiency.
- Pregnancy: Based on animal studies, may cause fetal harm.

Posology

- To be initiated 10 to 13 days prior to a scheduled procedure.
- Procedure must be initiated within 5 to 8 days of the last dose.
- To be taken orally with food once daily for 5 consecutive days.
- Dose varies according to the platelet count.

- *Platelet count*
  - $<40 \times 10^9$/L—60 mg OD
  - $>40 \times 10^9$/L—40 mg OD

Advantages

- Eltrombopag is a small molecule agonist towards c-mpl receptor (the physiological target of thrombopoietin). It has the risk of hepatotoxicity, and has restrictions with respect to the timing of specific types of food and drug administration.
- Romiplostim is a recombinant fusion protein analogue of thrombopoietin which is to be administered subcutaneously and causes bone marrow fibrosis.
- Avatrombopag can be administered orally with food, has no significant hepatotoxicity, it does not share the immunogenic and safety risks of the recombinant parenteral drugs.

Lusutrombopag

Thrombopoietic Receptor Agonist

Approval—July 31, 2018

Indication

Treatment of thrombocytopenia in adult patients with chronic liver disease scheduled to undergo a procedure

Mechanism of Action

- A small molecule TPO receptor agonist, Lusutrombopag, interacts with the transmembrane domain of human TPO receptors present on the megakaryocytes.
- The interaction stimulates proliferation and differentiation of the megakaryocytic progenitor cells from the hematopoietic stem cells and also promotes megakaryocyte maturation.

Pharmacokinetics

- Plasma protein binding is >99.9%.
- aVd is 39.5 L (healthy subjects).
- Metabolized by CYP4A11
- Primarily excreted in feces, 16% of which is unchanged.
- t½ is 27 hours.

Adverse Drug Reactions, Warnings and Precautions

- Headache frequently occurs.
- Thrombotic and thromboembolic complications are seen in patients with chronic liver disease.

Posology

- To be initiated 8 to 14 days prior to a scheduled procedure.
- The individual must undergo the procedure 2 to 8 days after the last dose.

Dose: 3 mg orally once daily with or without food for 7 days.

Advantages

- Lusutrombopag can be administered orally, has no significant risk of hepatotoxicity, and does not share immunogenic and safety concerns of recombinant parenteral molecules.

35

Fostamatinib Disodium Dehydrate

Tyrosine Kinase Inhibitor

Approval—April 17, 2018

Indication

Treatment of thrombocytopenia in chronic immune thrombo-cytopenia (ITP) patients with inadequate response to treatment

Mechanism of Action

- Fostamatinib and its active metabolite R406 inhibit Syk (a tyrosine kinase involved in the FcR signaling pathway).
- FcR on binding to its ligand causes phosphorylation of ITAM (immunoreceptor tyrosine-based activation motif) with the help of tyrosine kinases. This phosphorylation causes recruitment and downstream signaling that results in cytoskeletal rearrangement and phagocytosis.
- Thus, Fostamatinib and R406 inhibit Syk-dependent phagocytosis of autoantibody-coated platelets in patients with chronic ITP.

Pharmacokinetics

- It is a prodrug, metabolized in the gut by alkaline phosphatase to R406 (major metabolite, predominant systemic form) which is further metabolized by CYP3A4 and glucuronidation.
- t½ of R406 is 15 ($\pm$ 4.3).

Adverse Drug Reactions, Warnings and Precautions

- Common ADRs are diarrhea, hypertension, nausea, respiratory infection, dizziness, transaminase elevation, rash, abdominal pain, fatigue, chest pain and neutropenia.
- Embryo-fetal toxicity can occur.

Contraindications

- Pregnant and lactating women

Drug interactions

- Concomitant use with a strong CYP3A4 inhibitor increases exposure to R406.
- Use along with strong CYP3A4 inducers is not recommended.

Posology

100–150 mg orally twice daily.

Advantages

- Corticosteroids are the first line therapy. They inhibit Treg and B cell function, modulate FcR function. They are administered with or without IVIg and anti-D, which help impair antigen presentation and also competitively inhibit macrophage recognition of autoantibody-coated platelets.
- Second-line approach includes splenectomy and medical treatment with rituximab (which directly targets and depletes antibody-producing B cells) or TPO-RAs (stimulate megakaryocyte to produce new platelets).
- Despite the availability of therapies, there remains a significant amount of patients with relapsed or refractory disease having limited sensitivity to current approaches to treatment. Fostamatinib may prove to be beneficial in such situations.

4 | Drugs Acting on the Metabolic and Endocrine Systems

	Drug	Class	Indication
1	Burosumab-twza	Anti-FGF23 antibody	X-linked hypophosphatemia
2	Pegvaliase-pqpz	Phenylalanine ammonia lyase	Phenylketonuria
3	Ravulizumab-cwvz	Complement C5 inhibitor	Paroxysmal nocturnal hemoglobinuria
4	Sodium zirconium cyclosilicate	Potassium binder	Hyperkalemia
5	Elapegademase-lvlr	Adenosine deaminase	Adenosine Deaminase severe combined immune deficiency
6	Migalastat	Alpha galactosidase A	Fabry disease
7	Ethinyl estradiol and segesterone acetate	Vaginal contraceptive	Contraception
8	Elagolix	GnRH antagonist	Endometriosis

Burosumab-twza   Anti-FGF23 Antibody

Approval—April 17, 2018

Indication

Treatment of X-linked hypophosphatemia (XLH) in patients aged ≥1 year

Mechanism of Action

- X-linked hypophosphatemia is caused by an excess in fibroblast growth factor 23 (FGF23).
- FGF23 suppresses the renal tubular phosphate reabsorption and renal production of 1,25 dihydroxyvitamin D.
- Burosumab-twza, a recombinant human IgG1, anti-human FGF23 antibody, which binds to and inhibits the biological activity of FGF23, restoring the renal phosphate reabsorption as well as increasing the serum concentration of 1,25 dihydroxyvitamin D.

Pharmacokinetics

- Peaks at 8 to 11 days
- Follows first order kinetics
- aVd is 18L
- Metabolized by proteolysis
- t½ is 19 days.

Adverse Drug Reactions, Warnings and Precautions

- Children: Headache, injection site reaction, vomiting, pyrexia, extremity pain, decreased vitamin D.
- Adults: Backache, headache, tooth infection, restless leg syndrome, dizziness, constipation, reduced vitamin D, raised blood phosphorus.
- Hypersensitivity reactions may occur. Discontinue, if severe.
- Dose interruption or reduction may be needed in those who develop hyperphosphatemia and/or are at a risk of developing nephrocalcinosis.
- Cautious use in pregnant and lactating mothers.

Contraindications

- Coadministration with phosphate or active vitamin D analogues
- When phosphorus is within or above the normal range.
- Severe renal failure or ESRD (end stage renal disease)

Posology

As a subcutaneous injection

Pediatric dose:

- Starting dose: 0.8 mg/kg rounded to the nearest 10 mg, administered every two weeks. The minimum starting dose is 10 mg up to a maximum dose of 90 mg.
- Dose may be increased up to approximately 2 mg/kg (maximum 90 mg), administered every two weeks to achieve normal serum phosphorus.

Adult dose:

1 mg/kg body weight rounded to the nearest 10 mg up to a maximum dose of 90 mg administered every four weeks.

Advantages

- Reduced propensity to develop rickets in children.
- Fewer fractures in adults.

Pegvaliase-pqpz

Phenylalanine Ammonia Lyase

Approval—May 24, 2018

Indication

To reduce blood phenylalanine concentrations in adult patients with phenylketonuria (PKU), having uncontrolled blood phenylalanine concentrations (>600 micromol/L) on existing management

Mechanism of Action

- Pegvaliase-pqpz is a phenylalanine metabolizing enzyme, composed of recombinant phenylalanine ammonia lyase (rAvPAL) conjugated to N-hydroxysuccinimide (NHS)-methoxy-polyethylene glycol (PEG).
- PAL converts phenylalanine to ammonia and trans-cinnamic acid.
- Pegvaliase-pqpz acts as a substitute for the deficient phenylalanine hydroxylase (PAH) enzyme in patients with PKU and reduces the blood phenylalanine concentrations.

Pharmacokinetics

- Peaks at 8 hours
- Metabolized via catabolic pathways into small peptides and amino acids
- t½ is 47–60 hours.

Adverse Drug Reactions, Warnings and Precautions

Common ADRs are injection site reactions, arthralgia, hypersensitivity reactions, headache, generalized skin reactions lasting at least 14 days, pruritus, nausea, abdominal pain, oropharyngeal pain, vomiting, cough, diarrhea, fatigue.

Black Box Warning

Anaphylaxis may occur. Drug to be administered under supervision and patients to be observed closely for 1 hour. If self-administered, adrenaline should also be prescribed.

43

Contraindications

Pregnancy: Can cause fetal harm

Posology

- Initial dose—2.5 mg subcutaneously, once weekly for 4 weeks. To be titrated over 5 weeks, slowly.
- Increase the dose to a maximum of 40 mg SC OD in patients who have been on 20 mg OD continuously for at least 24 weeks and who have not achieved either a 20% reduction in blood phenylalanine concentration from pre-treatment baseline or a blood phenylalanine concentration ≤600/L.
- Discontinue in patients who have not achieved at least a 20% reduction in blood phenylalanine concentration from pre-treatment baseline or a blood phenylalanine concentration ≤600 micromol/L after 16 weeks of continuous treatment with the maximum dosage of 40 mg OD.
- Reduce the dosage and/or modify dietary protein and phenylalanine intake, as needed, to maintain blood phenylalanine concentrations within a clinically acceptable range and above 30/L.
- Monitor concentration of phenylalanine every 4 weeks.
- Pretreat to prevent hypersensitivity reactions.
- Rotate injection sites.

Advantages

- Response is seen within 4 weeks of therapy and is maintained.

Ravulizumab-cwvz

Complement C5 Inhibitor

Approval—December 21, 2018

Indication

Treatment of adult patients with paroxysmal nocturnal hemoglobinuria (PNH)

Mechanism of Action

- PNH is characterized by uncontrolled complement system activation.
- Ravulizumab-cwvz is a terminal complement inhibitor.
- It binds specifically and with high affinity to complement protein C5.
- It inhibits the cleavage of C5 to C5a and C5b and prevents the generation of the terminal complement complex C5b9, thus inhibiting the terminal complement-mediated intravascular hemolysis in patients with PNH.

Pharmacokinetics

t½ is 50 days.

Adverse Drug Reactions, Warnings and Precautions

- URTI and headache.
- Increased susceptibility to serious meningococcal infections. To be given only to individuals who have received meningococcal vaccination.
- Administered with caution in patients with any other systemic infection.
- Infusion reactions.

Contraindications

Unresolved *Neisseria meningitidis* infection.

Posology

Administered as an intravenous infusion, according to body weight, every 8 weeks.

- 40–60 kg: 2,400 mg followed by (f/b) 3000 mg
- 60–100 kg: 2700 mg f/b 3300 mg
- >100 kg: 3000 mg f/b 3600 mg

Advantages

- Eculizumab was the only approved complement inhibitor for PNH which needed to be administered every 2 weeks as an intravenous infusion.
- Ravulizumab is a new C5 inhibitor which shows immediate, complete, and sustained inhibition of complement protein C5 and has to be administered every 8 weeks.

Sodium Zirconium Cyclosilicate

Potassium Binder

Approval—April 18, 2018

Indication

Treatment of hyperkalemia, in adults

Mechanism of Action

- Non-absorbed zirconium silicate preferentially binds to potassium in exchange for hydrogen and sodium.
- It increases fecal potassium excretion by binding the potassium in the lumen of the gastrointestinal tract.
- Binding of potassium reduces the concentration of free potassium in the gastrointestinal lumen, reducing absorption and thereby lowering serum potassium levels.

Pharmacokinetics

- Organic, insoluble compound
- Not absorbed systemically
- Not metabolized
- Excreted in feces

Adverse Drug Reactions, Warnings and Precautions

- Mild to moderate edema. Monitoring is necessary, especially in patients who need to restrict their sodium intake or are prone to fluid overload.
- Gastrointestinal side effects occur, particularly in those with motility disorders.

Contraindications

None

Drug Interactions

- It causes an increase in the gastric pH and may interfere with the pH dependent absorption of drugs.
- Other oral medications should be administered at an interval of at least 2 hours, before or after.

Posology

⊕ 10 mg TDS, orally for up to 48 hours.

⊕ Maintenance: 10 mg OD, orally.

⊕ Adjust at 1 weekly intervals.

Limitations

⊕ Cannot be used as an emergency treatment for life-threatening hyperkalemia because of its delayed onset of action.

Elapegademase-lvlr   Adenosine Deaminase

Approval—October 5, 2018

Indication

Adenosine deaminase severe combined immune deficiency (ADA-SCID) in pediatric and adult patients

Mechanism of Action

- Elapegademase is a PEGylated recombinant adenosine deaminase (ADA) which acts as an exogenous source of ADA and leads to a reduction in the adenosine and deoxyadenosine nucleotide levels and an increase in the lymphocyte number.
- Deficiency of ADA is associated with SCID. ADA is involved in purine metabolism, catalyzing the irreversible hydrolytic deamination of adenosine or deoxyadenosine to inosine or deoxyinosine, respectively, as well as that of several other naturally occurring methylated adenosine compounds.
- Maintaining a low level of 2'-deoxyadenosine and adenosine is essential for maintaining a proper count number and function of immune cells as well as decreasing the frequency of opportunistic infections as an elevated adenosine level contributes to apoptosis and blocks the differentiation of thymocytes, causing severe T-lymphopenia.

Pharmacokinetics

- Peaks at 60 hours
- Metabolized by proteolysis

Adverse Drug Reactions, Warnings and Precautions

- Cough and vomiting are common.
- Anemia, thrombocytopenia, lymphoma, injection site erythema, urticaria are observed.
- Injection site bleeding may occur in patients with thrombocytopenia. Not to be used in those with severe thrombocytopenia.
- Delay in improvement of immune function can occur. Immunodeficient patients must be protected till immune function improves.

- To be avoided in pregnant and lactating mothers since studies are lacking.

Contraindications

None

Posology

- Transitioning from Pegademase—0.2 mg/kg weekly, intra-muscularly.
- Pegademase naïve—0.4 mg/kg weekly based on ideal body weight, divided into two doses (0.2 mg/kg twice a week), intramuscularly.

Limitations

- Paucity of data for pharmacokinetics, safety and efficacy, calls for more studies.

Migalastat Alpha-Galactosidase A

Approval—August 10, 2018

Indication

Treatment of adults with Fabry disease and an amenable galactosidase alpha gene (GLA) variant

Mechanism of Action

- Alpha-galactosidase A is encoded by the galactosidase alpha gene, GLA, which is deficient in Fabry disease.
- Migalastat is a chaperone that reversibly binds to the active site of the alpha-galactosidase A (alpha-Gal A).
- The binding stabilizes alpha-Gal A allowing its trafficking from the endoplasmic reticulum into the lysosome where it exerts its action.
- In the lysosome, at a lower pH and at a higher concentration of substrates, migalastat dissociates from alpha-Gal A allowing it to breakdown the glycosphingolipids, globotriaosylceramide (GL-3) and globotriaosylsphingosine (lyso-Gb3).
- Certain GLA variants causing Fabry disease result in the production of abnormally folded, less stable forms of the alpha-Gal-A which retain enzymatic activity. These amenable GLA variants produce alpha-Gal A proteins that may be stabilized by migalastat thereby restoring their trafficking to lysosomes and their intralysosomal activity.

Pharmacokinetics

- Peaks at 3 hours
- Oral bioavailability is 75%.
- Food reduces absorption.
- aVd is 87 L
- Metabolized by uridine diphosphate glucuronosyltransferase (UDPGT)
- Excreted in feces
- t½ is 4 hours.

Adverse Drug Reactions, Warnings and Precautions

- Common ADRs are headache, cough, nasopharyngitis, UTIs, nausea, pyrexia, epistaxis.

Contraindications

None

Posology

- 123 mg orally once every alternate day at the same time of day, on empty stomach.
- Food should not be consumed for 2 hours at least.
- Drug should not be administered on 2 consecutive days.
- If a dose is missed entirely for the day, the missed dose is administered only if it is within 12 hours of the normal time that the dose should have been taken. If more than 12 hours have passed, administer the next planned dose according to the every-other-day dosing schedule.

Ethinyl Estradiol and Segesterone Acetate

Vaginal Contraceptive

Approval—August 10, 2018

Indication

As a vaginal contraceptive

Mechanism of Action

Suppression of ovulation

Pharmacokinetics

⊕ Peaks at 2 hours

Segesterone acetate (SA):
- aVd is 19.6 L.
- 95% plasma protein bound
- t½ is 4.5 hours.

Ethinyl estradiol (EE):
- 85.5% plasma protein bound
- Causes an increase in the serum concentration of sex hormone binding globulin.
- t½ is 15.1 hours, undergoes enterohepatic circulation.

⊕ Metabolized by CYP3A4; EE also undergoes aromatic hydroxylation, methylation, glucuronidation and sulfate conjugation; metabolites have weak estrogenic activity.

Adverse Drug Reactions, Warnings and Precautions

⊕ Common ADRs are headache, migraine, nausea, vomiting, vulvovaginal fungal infections, abdominal pain, dysmenorrhea, vaginal discharge, UTIs, breast discomfort and tenderness, bleeding irregularities including menorrhagia, diarrhea, genital pruritus.

⊕ Stop the drug 4 weeks before to 2 weeks after a major surgery, as chances of thrombotic phenomena increase. Stop if a thromboembolic event occurs.

⊕ Administer only after 4 weeks of delivery, in mothers who are not breastfeeding.

- Assess cardiovascular risk factors in all women, especially those >35 years.
- Stop, if jaundice occurs.
- In those with controlled hypertension, monitor blood pressure. Avoid in women with uncontrolled hypertension or hypertension with a vascular disease.
- Monitor glucose and lipid levels. Use an alternative method of contraception, if those with uncontrolled dyslipidemias or diabetes.
- Assess changes in headache, discontinue, if required.
- Can cause amenorrhea. Evaluate, if bleeding irregularities persist.
- Discontinue, if pregnancy occurs.
- Avoid in lactating mothers as it can decrease milk production.

Contraindications

- High risk of arterial or venous thrombotic diseases
- Current or history of estrogen and/or progesterone sensitive breast cancer
- Liver diseases
- Undiagnosed uterine bleeding
- Use of Hepatitis C drug combinations containing ombitasvir, paritaprevir or ritonavir, with or without dasabuvir, as liver enzymes increase. Use the system only after 2 weeks of stopping anti-HCV therapy.
- Hypersensitivity to the components of the ring

Drug Interactions

CYP3A4 inducers may decrease effectiveness or increase breakthrough bleeding. Alternative method of contraception should be used in such situations.

Posology

- A silicone elastomer vaginal system containing 103 mg of segesterone acetate and 17.4 mg of ethinyl estradiol; releases, on an average, 0.15 mg/day of SA and 0.013 mg/day of EE.
- Has to be inserted vaginally and kept in place for 3 weeks followed by 1 week off.
- One system provides contraception for 13 28-day cycles.

Advantages

- Has to be applied locally.
- Effect lasts for a year.

Limitations

- Not adequately evaluated in women with BMI >29 kg/m^2.

Elagolix

GnRH Antagonist

Approval—April 17, 2018

Indication

Treatment of moderate to severe pain associated with endometriosis

Mechanism of Action

- Elagolix is a competitive GnRH receptor antagonist. It binds to the GnRH receptors in the pituitary gland and inhibits endogenous GnRH signaling.
- The binding results in a dose dependent suppression of LH and FSH, in turn reducing the blood levels of estradiol and progesterone.

Pharmacokinetics

- Peaks at 1 hour
- 80% plasma protein bound
- Metabolized by CYP3A4 (major), CYP2D6, CYP2C8, UGTs (minor)
- Excreted in feces
- $t\frac{1}{2}$ is 4–6 hours.

Adverse Drug Reactions, Warnings and Precautions

- Hot flushes, night sweats, headache, nausea, insomnia, amenorrhea, anxiety, arthralgia, depression, and mood changes are common.
- Bone loss may occur. Assess bone mineral density in women with additional risk factors for bone loss.
- Alteration of menstrual bleeding may make detection of pregnancy difficult. Discontinue, if pregnancy occurs.
- New onset or worsening of mood disorders can occur.
- Hepatic transaminases may rise.
- May reduce efficacy of concomitant estrogen-containing contraceptive. Non-hormonal contraceptive should be used during and till 1 week after treatment with Elagolix.

Contraindications

- Pregnancy
- Known osteoporosis
- Severe hepatic impairment
- With concomitant strong OATP1B1 inhibitors

Drug Interactions

- A moderate inducer of CYP3A, decreases plasma concentration of substrates.
- Inhibitor of P-gp, increases plasma concentration of substrates.
- A substrate of CYP3A, P-gp, and OATP1B1. Interactions with inducers and inhibitors can occur.

Posology

- Normal liver function or mild hepatic impairment—150 mg OD for up to 24 months or 200 mg BD for up to 6 months, orally.
- Moderate liver impairment—150 mg OD for up to 6 months, orally.

Advantages

- Oral treatment ensures better compliance.

5 Drugs Acting on the Eye

	Drug	Class	Indication
1.	Cenegermin-bkbj	Nerve growth factor	Neurotrophic keratitis
2.	Loteprednol etabonate	Corticosteroid	Postoperative ocular pain and inflammation

Cenegermin-bkbj | Nerve Growth Factor

Approval—August 22, 2018

Indication

Treatment of neurotrophic keratitis in adults, moderate (persistent epithelial defect) to severe (corneal ulcer)

Mechanism of Action

Cenegermin bkbj is a recombinant human nerve growth factor which acts through specific high-affinity (i.e. TrkA) and low-affinity (i.e. p75NTR) nerve growth factor receptors in the anterior segment of the eye to support corneal innervation and integrity.

Pharmacokinetics

- Removed from the eye via tears and the nasolacrimal duct, majorly.
- No systemic absorption occurs.
- Distributes mostly to the anterior chamber.
- Though not systemically absorbed, caution is to be exercised when administered to pregnant or lactating women.

Adverse Drug Reactions, Warnings and Precautions

- Common ADRs are eye pain, ocular hyperemia, eye inflammation, increased lacrimation.
- Contact lenses should be removed before administration and be reinserted only after 15 minutes.

Contraindications

None

Posology

- One drop in the affected eye, 6 times a day, at 2 hour intervals, for 8 weeks.
- If more than one topical ophthalmic product is used, an interval of 15 minutes is to be maintained.

Advantages

⊕ Complete corneal healing occurs in most patients within 8 weeks, compared to placebo.

⊕ Can be used in children above 2 years of age.

⊕ No dose modification is needed in the elderly.

Loteprednol Etabonate   Corticosteroid

Approval—August 22, 2018

Indication

Post-ocular surgery pain and inflammation

Mechanism of action

- Loteprednol etabonate acts as an anti-inflammatory agent.
- It inhibits edema, fibrin deposition, capillary dilation, leukocyte migration, capillary proliferation, fibroblast proliferation, deposition of collagen, and scar formation associated with inflammation.

Pharmacokinetics

- Lipid soluble, enters cells
- Extensively metabolized into inactive metabolites

Adverse Drug Reactions, Warnings and Precautions

- Common ADRs are anterior chamber inflammation, eye pain, foreign body sensation.
- Prolonged use may result in a rise in the intraocular pressure and glaucoma, damage to the optic nerve, visual acuity and field defects. Monitor, if used beyond 10 days.
- Posterior subcapsular cataract may occur.
- Delayed wound healing and bleb formation is a possibility. Perforation may occur in the diseases causing corneal thinning. Monitor when necessary.
- Infections, bacterial, viral or fungal, may exacerbate.

Contraindications

- Viral diseases of the cornea and conjunctiva including epithelial herpes simplex keratitis (dendritic keratitis), vaccinia, and varicella, mycobacterial or fungal infection of the eye
- Pregnancy category C
- Caution while administering to a lactating woman

63

Posology

1 to 2 drops in the conjunctival sac of the affected eye 4 times a day beginning the day after surgery, through 2 weeks postoperatively.

Limitations

⊕ All limitations of corticosteroids also apply to this drug.

6 Drugs Acting on the Musculoskeletal System

	Drug	Class	Indication
1	Baricitinib	JAK inhibitor	Rheumatoid arthritis
2	Amifampridine phosphate	Potassium channel blocker	Lambert-Eaton myasthenic syndrome

Baricitinib | JAK Inhibitor

Approval—May 31, 2018

Indication

Treatment of adult patients with moderate to severely active rheumatoid arthritis, who have had an inadequate response to one or more TNF antagonist therapies

Mechanism of Action

- Baricitinib is a Janus kinase (JAK) inhibitor with greater inhibitory potency at JAK1, JAK2 and TYK2 as compared to JAK3.
- JAKs are intracellular enzymes which transmit signals arising from cytokine/growth factor-receptor interactions on the cellular membrane to influence cellular processes of hematopoiesis and immune cell function.
- In the signaling pathway, they phosphorylate and activate signal transducers and activators of transcription (STATs) which modulate intracellular activity including gene expression.
- Baricitinib modulates the signaling pathway at the level of JAKs, thereby preventing the phosphorylation and activation of STATs.

Pharmacokinetics

- Peaks at 1 hour
- Steady state at 2–3 days
- Absolute bioavailability is 80%.
- Food reduces absorption.
- aVd is 76 L.
- 50% plasma protein bound
- Substrate of P-gp, BCRP, OAT3 and MATE2-K transporters
- Metabolized by CYP3A4
- Excreted in urine
- t½ is 12 hours.

Adverse Drug Reactions, Warnings and Precautions

- Common ADRs are URTIs, nausea, herpes simplex, herpes zoster.
- Serious infections, including localized infections, may occur.

Interruption of the drug and treatment of the infection should be initiated.

⊕ Cautious use in those at a risk of thrombosis or gastrointestinal perforations.

⊕ Cell counts may drop. Monitoring is recommended.

⊕ Avoid use with live vaccines, in pregnant and lactating mothers.

Black Box Warning

⊕ Serious infections, including tuberculosis, bacterial, invasive fungal, viral and/or other opportunistic infections leading to hospitalization or death may occur.

⊕ Lymphoma and other malignancies may occur.

⊕ Thrombosis, including deep venous thrombosis, pulmonary embolism, and arterial thrombosis, sometimes fatal, may occur.

Contraindications

None

Drug Interactions

⊕ Should not be used concomitantly with drugs acting on OAT3 transporters like probenecid.

Posology

⊕ 2 mg OD, orally; as monotherapy or in combination with methotrexate or other DMARDS.

⊕ Avoid initiation or discontinue, if HB <8 g/dL or absolute lymphocyte count is <500 cells/mm^3 or absolute neutrophil count is <1000 cells/mm^3.

⊕ Not recommended in patients with severe hepatic or moderate to severe renal impairment.

Limitations

⊕ Cannot be used concomitantly with other JAK inhibitors, biologic DMARDs, or potent immunosuppressants such as azathioprine, cyclosporine.

Amifampridine Phosphate

Potassium Channel Blocker

Approval—November 28, 2018

Indication

Treatment of Lambert-Eaton myasthenic syndrome (LEMS) in adult patients

Mechanism of Action

- Amifampridine phosphate is a broad-spectrum potassium channel blocker.
- It prolongs cell depolarization, thus allowing more influx of calcium into nerve endings.
- This facilitates release of acetylcholine from vesicles and enhances transmission of impulse.

Pharmacokinetics

- t½ is 1.8–2.5 hours.
- Extensively metabolized by N-acetyltransferase
- 90–100% eliminated via urine.

Adverse Drug Reactions, Warnings and Precautions

The common ADRs seen are paresthesia, respiratory infections, pain in abdomen, nausea, diarrhea, headache, raised liver enzymes, backache, hypertension, muscular spasms, seizures, hypersensitivity reactions.

Contraindications

- History of seizures
- Uncontrolled asthma
- Concomitant use with drugs having narrow therapeutic index
- Concomitant use with drugs causing QTc prolongation
- In patients with congenital QT syndromes
- Hypersensitivity to amifampridine or another aminopyridine

Drug Interactions

- Concomitant use with drugs that lower seizure threshold may lead to an increased risk of seizures.
- Concomitant use with drugs having cholinergic effects may increase the risk of cholinergic adverse reactions.

Posology

- 15–30 mg daily taken orally in divided doses (3 to 4 times daily).
- Should not be used in pregnancy, as it may cause fetal harm.
- Use with caution in patients having hepatic or renal impairment.

Advantages

- Amifampridine (3,4 diaminopyridine) is a first-line drug for symptomatic treatment for LEMS. Approved for use in LEMS by the European Medicines Agency in 2009.
- However, there are issues concerning its batch-batch variation in quality and potency and possibility of compounding errors which risks the patient to under or over dosing.
- The phosphate salt form of amifampridine is more stable compared to its base form.
- Fampridine (a 4-aminopyridine, was earlier used for LEMS) is more neurotoxic and less potent than amifampridine.

7 Drugs Acting on the Skin

	Drug	Class	Indication
1.	Tildrakizumab - asmn	IL-23 antagonist	Plaque psoriasis

Tildrakizumab-asmn

IL-23 Antagonist

Approval—March 20, 2018

Indication

Treatment of moderate-to-severe plaque psoriasis in adult candidates of systemic therapy or phototherapy

Mechanism of Action

- Tildrakizumab-asmn is a humanized IgG1/k antibody that binds to the p19 subunit of interleukin-23 (IL-23), an inflammatory cytokine, and inhibits its interaction with IL-23 receptor, thus preventing the release of proinflammatory cytokines and chemokines.

Pharmacokinetics

- Peaks at 6 days
- Absolute bioavailability is 73–80%
- aVd is 10.8 L.
- Metabolized proteolytically
- t½ is 23 days.

Adverse Drug Reactions, Warnings and Precautions

- URTIs, injection site reactions, diarrhea are common.
- Serious hypersensitivity reactions may warrant discontinuation.
- Risk of infection, including tuberculosis, increases. Evaluation before, during and after therapy is a must.
- Caution must be practiced, if administered in pregnant or lactating mothers.

Contraindications

Hypersensitivity to any component of the product

Drug Interactions

- Live vaccines should not be administered concomitantly.
- Increases the plasma concentration of drugs metabolized by CYP2D6.

Posology

100 mg at weeks 0, 4 and every 12 weeks thereafter, subcutaneously.

Advantages

⊕ Good response is observed after regular treatment for at least 12 weeks, and is much more if therapy is continued further.

8 Drugs Acting on the Gastrointestinal System

	Drug	Class	Indication
1	Polyethylene glycol 3350 with electrolytes	Osmotic laxative	Colon cleansing in colonoscopy
2	Fosnetupitant/ Palonosetron	Antiemetic	Chemotherapy-induced nausea and vomiting

Polyethylene Glycol (PEG) 3350 with Electrolytes

Osmotic Laxative

Approval—May 7, 2018

Indication

Colon cleansing for colonoscopy, in adults

Mechanism of Action

- PEG-3350 is an oral solution comprising of polyethylene glycol 3350, sodium ascorbate, sodium sulfate, ascorbic acid, sodium chloride and potassium chloride.
- The unabsorbed PEG, ascorbate and sulfate exert an osmotic effect in the gastrointestinal tract, thus producing copious watery diarrhea.
- The first bowel movement occurs about 1–2 hours after the onset of therapy.

Pharmacokinetics

t½ are:
- PEG—4 hours
- Ascorbate—7 hours
- Sulfate—10 hours

Adverse Drug Reactions, Warnings and Precautions

- Bloating, dyspepsia, abdominal pain and distension, vomiting, dizziness, and sleep disorders are common. Fluid and electrolyte abnormalities, cardiac arrhythmias, seizures, colonic mucosal ulceration, ischemic colitis and ulcerative colitis may occur.
- PEG may cause hypersensitivity reactions.
- Should be used with caution in patients with renal insufficiency; adequate hydration should be maintained.

Special Instructions

- Consumption of clear liquids only, from the onset of therapy until after the colonoscopy.

- No other laxative should be consumed.
- No oral medication should be consumed 1 hour before or after each dose.
- Completion of dose 2, including all additional liquids, at least 2 hours before the colonoscopy must be ensured.

Contraindications

Gastrointestinal obstruction, perforated bowel, gastric retention, ileus, toxic megacolon, hypersensitivity to any of the components

Drug Interactions

- Reduces the absorption of co-administered drugs.
- Increases the risk of mucosal ulceration and ischemic colitis when given with stimulant laxatives.

Posology

- 2 doses are required.
- Dose 1: PEG 3350 plus sodium sulfate.
- Dose 2: Sodium ascorbate and ascorbic acid plus PEG-3350.
- 2-day dosing and 1 day dosing regimen can be followed.
- Interval of at least 2 hours between the 2 doses must be maintained.

Advantages

- PEG-3350 has a low total volume (1L), thus improving patient colonoscopy preparation experience; as high volume bowel preparations are troublesome due to large volumes and unpleasant taste.
- Offers whole bowel cleansing with an additional focus on the ascending colon.

Fosnetupitant/ Palonosetron

Antiemetic

Approval—April 19, 2018

Indication

In combination with dexamethasone to prevent acute and delayed nausea and vomiting associated with initial and repeat courses of highly emetogenic cancer chemotherapy in adults

Mechanism of Action

- Fosnetupitant—NK1 receptor antagonist which prevents nausea, vomiting in both acute and delayed phase.
- Palonosetron, on the other hand, is a 5-HT_3 antagonist which prevents nausea, vomiting only during the acute phase.

Pharmacokinetics

Fosnetupitant:
- Prodrug, converted to netupitant by hydrolysis.
- Metabolized by CYP3A4 (major), CYP2C9, 2D6 (minor) to form active metabolites M1,2,3
- Excreted via feces primarily
- t½ is 0.75 $\pm$ 0.4 hours; Netupitant: 144 $\pm$ 73 hours

Palonosetron:
- 50% metabolized to relatively inactive metabolite by CYP2D6, 3A4, 1A2
- Excreted via urine, 40% unchanged
- t½ is 58 $\pm$ 27 hours

Adverse Drug Reactions, Warnings and Precautions

- Headache, asthenia, dyspepsia, fatigue, constipation, erythema, hypersensitivity reactions, serotonin syndrome may occur.

Contraindications

- Pregnancy: May cause fetal harm
- Severe hepatic and renal impairment

Drug Interactions

- Netupitant inhibits CYP3A4 and increases plasma concentrations of its substrates given concomitantly for up to 6 days after a single dose. Hence, concomitant CYP3A4 substrates should be avoided for a week, in unavoidable cases, dose reduction of the substrate should be considered.
- CYP3A4 inducers (e.g. rifampin) decrease its plasma concentration.

Posology

235 mg Fosnetupitant with 0.25 mg Palonosetron lyophilized powder reconstituted in 50 mL of 5% dextrose injection or 0.9% sodium chloride (normal saline) injection and administered as 30-minute infusion approximately 30 minutes prior to the start of chemotherapy.

Limitations

Not been studied for the prevention of nausea and vomiting associated with anthracycline-cyclophosphamide chemotherapy.

9 | Anti-Infective Drugs

	Drug	Class	Indication
1	Doravirine	NNRTI	HIV-1 infection
2	Bictegravir/emtricitabine/tenofovir alafenamide	Antiretroviral	HIV-1 infection
3	Ibalizumab-uiyk	CD4 post attachment inhibitor	HIV-1 infection
4	Baloxavir marboxil	Anti-influenza	Symptomatic uncomplicated influenza
5	Tecovirimat	Antiviral	Smallpox
6.	Sarecycline	Tetracycline antibiotic	Acne vulgaris
7.	Omadacycline	Tetracycline antibiotic	Community acquired bacterial pneumonia; Acute bacterial skin and structure infections
8.	Eravacycline	Tetracycline antibiotic	Intra-abdominal infections
9.	Plazomicin	Aminoglycoside antibiotic	Complicated UTI
10.	Tafenoquine	Antimalarial	Vivax malaria
11.	Moxidectin	Anthelmintic	Onchocerciasis

Doravirine

Antiretroviral NNRTI

Approval—August 30, 2018

Indication

Treatment of HIV-1 infection in combination with other antiretroviral drugs in adult, treatment naive patient

Mechanism of Action

Doravirine is an antiretroviral drug that acts as a non-competitive, non-nucleoside reverse transcriptase inhibitor (NNRTI) active against HIV-1 virus.

Pharmacokinetics

- 64% oral bioavailability
- 76% protein binding
- Metabolized by CYP3A
- Extensively metabolized
- Excreted unchanged in urine—6%, unchanged in feces—minor
- t½ is 15 hours.

Adverse Drug Reactions, Warnings and Precautions

Common ADRs experienced are nausea, dizziness, diarrhea, headache, fatigue, pain in abdomen, abnormal dreams, immune reconstitution syndrome.

Contraindications

- Strong CYP3A4 inducers: Decrease the plasma concentration and hence the effectiveness. A 4-week cessation period is recommended prior to initiation of doravirine.
- Combination with efavirenz, etravirine and nevirapine

Drug Interactions

Interacts with CYP3A inducers (e.g. rifabutin) and inhibitors (e.g. ketoconazole).

Posology

- 100 mg orally once daily.
- With Rifabutin: One tablet BD.
- No dose adjustment required in mild-to-severe renal or mild-to-moderate hepatic impairment. It has not been studied in patients on dialysis and those having severe hepatic impairment.

Advantages

- It can be prescribed as a once-daily medication alone or with tenofovir disoproxil fumarate and lamivudine as a single pill.
- It is active *in vitro* against a wide range of viruses that show transmitted NNRTI-resistance-associated mutations.
- Antiviral efficacy of combination regimens with DOR was found to be non-inferior compared to ritonavir-boosted darunavir or EFV in treatment-naïve patients and in patients with high-plasma viral loads.
- As compared to EFV, it has a better safety profile. Patients on DOR experience less neuropsychiatric and cutaneous adverse events.
- DOR is now being investigated in treatment-experienced patients and in those with transmitted NNRTI drug resistance.

Bictegravir/ Emtricitabine/ Tenofovir Alafenamide — Antiretroviral FDDC

Approval—February 7, 2018

Indication

Treatment of HIV-1 infection in treatment naïve or virologically suppressed adults (HIV-1 RNA <50 copies per mL) on a stable antiretroviral regimen for at least 3 months without history of treatment failure and known substitutions associated with resistance to the individual components of the FDDC

Mechanism of Action

- Three-drug combination: Bictegravir 50 mg (BIC), emtricitabine (FTC) 200 mg and tenofovir alafenamide (TAF) 25 mg.
- BIC is a novel HIV-1 integrase strand transfer inhibitor (INSTI). It blocks the action of HIV integrase that catalyzes two consecutive reactions required to facilitate insertion of the reverse-transcribed viral genome into the host genome, viz. 3′processing of the viral DNA and strand transfer.
- Emtricitabine and Tenofovir alafenamide are nucleoside reverse transcriptase inhibtors (NRTIs).

Pharmacokinetics

	BIC	FTC	TAF
t½ (hours)	17	10	0.5
Elimination	CYP3A UGT1A1	Renal	Cathepsin A, CES1 (hepatocytes)
Excretion in feces and urine (%)	60 and 35	13 and 70	31 and < 1

Adverse Drug Reactions, Warnings and Precautions

- Common ADRs seen are diarrhea, nausea, and headache.
- Immune reconstitution syndrome may occur.
- New onset or worsening renal impairment, lactic acidosis/severe hepatomegaly with steatosis have been observed.

⊕ Prior to initiation, screening for hepatitis B virus infection is required as severe acute exacerbations of hepatitis B have been experienced in co-infected patients who have discontinued emtricitabine or tenofovir containing medications.

Contraindications

Co-administration with dofetilide and rifampin

Drug Interactions

⊕ Since it is a complete regimen, co-administration with other antiretroviral drugs is not recommended.
⊕ When co-administered with dofetilide, its plasma concentration increases while rifampin decreases BIC plasma concentrations, may result in the loss of efficacy and development of resistance.

Dose

⊕ One tablet, once daily with or without food.
⊕ Not recommended in patients with estimated creatinine clearance < 30 mL/min, severe hepatic impairment.

Ibalizumab-uiyk

CD4 Post Attachment Inhibitor

Approval—March 6, 2018

Indication

Treatment of adults with multidrug resistant HIV-1 infection, failing current antiretroviral regimen

Mechanism of Action

- Ibalizumab is a recombinant humanized IgG-4 monoclonal antibody.
- It binds to surface domain 2 on the CD4 cells and prevents conformational changes in the CD4–HIV envelope glycoprotein (gp120) complex, which is required for virus entry into host cells.
- Since domain 1 is spared for binding to MHC II, immunosuppression does not occur.

Pharmacokinetics

- t½ is 3.3 days.

Adverse Drug Reactions, Warnings and Precautions

- Common ADRs are diarrhea, dizziness, nausea and rash.
- Immune reconstitution inflammatory syndrome may occur.

Contraindications

None

Drug Interactions

None

Posology

- Intravenously as a single loading dose of 2 g
- Followed by a maintenance dose of 800 mg every 2 weeks after dilution in 250 mL of 0.9% NaCl

Advantages

⊕ Ibalizumab also acts on CCR5- and CXCR4-tropic strains as it targets HIV-1 entry before coreceptor binding and fusion have taken place.

⊕ Based on the mechanism of action and target-mediated drug disposition, drug interactions are not expected.

⊕ There is no evidence to suggest cross-resistance with other antiretroviral drugs.

⊕ It is superior in potency and spectrum of activity against HIV-1 virus isolates as compared to the neutralising monoclonal antibodies currently under clinical development.

Limitations

⊕ It carries a risk for immunogenicity.

⊕ Safety and efficacy in pediatric and geriatric population has not been established.

Baloxavir Marboxil | Anti-Influenza

Approval—October 24, 2018

Indication

Treatment of acute uncomplicated influenza in patients symptomatic for <48 hours

Mechanism of action

- Cap snatching is required by the virus to hijack the host mRNA transcription system to facilitate viral RNA synthesis.
- Baloxavir marboxil inhibits cap snatching by inhibiting cap-endonuclease, thereby inhibiting replication activity of the viral polymerase.

Pharmacokinetics

- Prodrug, converted to Baloxavir (active metabolite)
- Protein bound: 92.9–93.9%
- Metabolized by UGT1A3 (major) and CYP3A4 (minor)
- Excreted primarily via feces
- t½ is 79.1 hours.

Adverse Drug Reactions, Warnings and Precautions

- Common ADRs are diarrhea, bronchitis, nausea, nasopharyngitis, headache.
- No adverse developmental effects observed in rats or rabbits exposed to 5 to 7 times the maximal recommended human dose, however, Baloxavir and its metabolites were present in milk of lactating rats. Studies in humans are lacking.

Contraindications

Hypersensitivity to the drug or any of its components

Drug Interactions

- Forms chelates with polyvalent cations such as calcium, aluminum, magnesium in food or medication and retards their absorption.

⊕ Co-administration with live-attenuated influenza vaccine (LAIV) may inhibit the viral replication of the vaccine and cause reduction in its effectiveness.

Posology

Route: Oral
Dose: Single dose
40 to <80 kg: 40 mg, ≥80 kg: 80 mg

Advantages

⊕ It acts via a novel mechanism, which makes it active against viruses that are resistant to other drugs as well.

Limitations

⊕ Influenza viruses change with time and factors (e.g. virus type or subtype, emergence of resistance, changes in viral virulence) which makes it necessary to check for drug susceptibility patterns for circulating influenza virus strains before initiating treatment.

Tecovirimat | Antiviral

Approval—July 13, 2018

Indication

Treatment of human smallpox disease in adults and pediatric patients weighing ≥13 kg

Mechanism of Action

- Inhibits the orthopoxvirus VP37 envelope wrapping protein
- Prevents the formation and egress of enveloped virions vital for virulence.

Pharmacokinetics

- Metabolized by hydrolysis, UGT1A1and 1A4
- Excreted in urine (73%) and feces (23% unchanged)
- t½ is 20 hours.

Adverse Drug Reactions, Warnings and Precautions

- Headache, nausea, abdominal pain, and vomiting are the common ADRs.

Drug Interactions

- Weak CYP3A inducer, CYP2C8 and 2C19 inhibitor.
- Co-administration with Repaglinide may cause hypoglycemia.
- Decreases plasma concentration of midazolam.
- Co-administration with live smallpox vaccine may reduce the immune response to the vaccine.

Posology

To be taken twice daily for 14 days, within 30 minutes of a fatty meal.
- Adults: 600 mg
- Pediatric patients:
    - 13 – <25 kg: 200 mg
    - 25 – <40 kg: 400 mg
    - ≥40 kg: 600 mg

Advantages

- Though eradicated in 1980, the causative agent for smallpox persists and could be used as a bioweapon.
- The smallpox vaccine is no longer used in the general population, herd immunity is minimal and the vaccine is ineffective after the onset of clinical illness.
- Hence, Tecovirimat could act as an important measure for the treatment of clinical disease until standard vaccine can be effectively deployed.

Limitations

- Human trials for smallpox were not feasible because inducing the disease in humans would be unethical hence, its effectiveness was established based only on results efficacy studies conducted in non-human primates and rabbits infected with non-variola orthopoxvirus.
- Its efficacy may be reduced in immunocompromised patients.

Sarecycline

Tetracycline Antibiotic

Approval—October 1, 2018

Indication

Treatment of inflammatory non-nodular moderate to severe acne vulgaris, in patients ≥9 years of age

Mechanism of Action

- Similar to the older tetracyclines, Sarecycline, by binding to the 30S ribosomes, prevents protein synthesis.
- *Antimicrobial spectrum:* Effective against acne-specific pathogens, viz., *Propionibacterium acnes, Staphylococcus aureus.*

Pharmacokinetics

- Plasma protein binding—62–74%
- Minimal hepatic metabolism
- Excreted in feces and urine
- t½ is 21–22 hours.

Adverse Drug Reactions, Warnings and Precautions

- Common ADRs are nausea, teeth discoloration when given during teeth development, antibiotic associated colitis (less than doxycycline and minocycline), photosensitivity.
- CNS side effects like dizziness, vertigo can occur; should be cautioned about driving and using hazardous machinery.

Contraindications

- Pregnancy and lactation
- Hypersensitivity to tetracycline

Drug Interactions

- Increased risk of raised intracranial pressure with oral retinoids.
- Antacids and iron preparations impair absorption.
- It interferes with bactericidal action of penicillin.

- Depresses plasma prothrombin time, greater risk of bleeding with anticoagulants.
- Increases levels of Pg-p substrates (e.g. digoxin).

Posology

- Once daily orally with or without food.
  To be swallowed with adequate amounts of fluid to reduce risk of esophageal irritation or ulceration.
- *Dose:*
  60 mg: 33–54 kg
  100 mg: 55–84 kg
  150 mg: 85–136 kg

Advantages

- Narrow spectrum tetracycline antibiotic with limited activity against aerobic gram-negative gastrointestinal organisms as compared to minocycline and doxycycline, hence lesser potential of causing superinfections.

Limitations

- Efficacy beyond 12 weeks and safety beyond 12 months of administration has not been established.

Omadacycline

Tetracycline Antibiotic

Approval—October 2, 2018

Indications

- Community-acquired bacterial pneumonia (CABP)
- Acute bacterial skin and skin structure infections (ABSSSI)

Mechanism of Action

- Binds to the 30S ribosomal subunit and blocks protein synthesis.
- Broad spectrum, bacteriostatic.
- Bactericidal against few *S. pneumoniae* and *H. influenzae* isolates.

Pharmacokinetics

- Oral bioavailability is 34.5%.
- Not metabolized
- 81% eliminated in feces
- t½ is 13–16 hours.

Adverse Drug Reactions, Warnings and Precautions

- Nausea, vomiting, infusion site reactions, raised serum transaminases and gamma-glutamyl transferase, hypertension, headache, diarrhea, insomnia, and constipation are the most frequent ADRs.
- Tooth discoloration and enamel hypoplasia can occur.
- The use during the second and third trimesters of pregnancy, infancy and childhood up to the age of 8 years may cause reversible inhibition of bone growth.
- *Clostridium difficile*-associated diarrhea, photosensitivity, pseudotumor cerebri may occur.
- Anti-anabolic action causes increased BUN (blood urea nitrogen), azotemia, acidosis, hyperphosphatemia, pancreatitis and abnormal liver function.

Drug Interactions

- Dose of anticoagulants needs to be decreased.

- Absorption is impaired by antacids containing aluminum, calcium, or magnesium, bismuth subsalicylate and iron containing preparations.

Posology

- Treatment duration: 7–14 days.
- Fasting of minimum 4 hours before taking oral tablets.

	Loading dose	Maintenance dose
Oral use	450 mg OD for 2 days	300 mg OD
IV infusion	200 mg over 60 minutes	100 mg over 30 minutes
	OR 100 mg over 30 minutes	OR 300 mg oral OD

Advantages

- No dose adjustment is required in hepatic or renal impairment.
- Aminomethylcycline structure makes it unique:
  - Helps overcome bacterial resistance due to efflux pumps and ribosomal protection.
  - Increases antimicrobial potency.
  - Causes less nausea and vomiting as compared to tigecycline.

Eravacycline

Tetracycline Antibiotic

Approval—August 27, 2018

Indication

Treatment of complicated intra-abdominal infection in patients >18 years of age

Mechanism of Action

Binds to the 30S ribosomal subunit and prevents the incorporation of amino acid residues into the elongating peptide chains.

Pharmacokinetics

- Metabolized by CYP3A4 and FMO mediated oxidation
- 34% excreted in urine and 47% in feces as unchanged and 20% in urine and 17% in feces as metabolites
- t½ is 20 hours.

Adverse Drug Reactions, Warnings and Precautions

- Life-threatening allergic reactions, *Clostridium difficile*-associated diarrhea may occur.
- Permanent teeth discoloration (yellow-gray-brown), enamel hypoplasia, and reversible inhibition of bone growth occurs when administered during the second and third trimesters of pregnancy, infancy up to the age of 8 years.
- Women should not breastfeed during treatment.

Mechanism of Resistance

- Upregulation of non-specific intrinsic multi-drug-resistant (MDR) efflux
- Target-site modification

Drug Interactions

- Strong CYP3A inducers decrease the exposure of eravacycline (increase the dose).
- Those on anticoagulant therapy may require lowering of the anticoagulant dose.

Posology

1 mg/kg by IV infusion over 1 hour every 12 hours for a total duration of 4 to 14 days.

Advantages

⊕ Novel, synthetic fluorocycline antibiotic, with *in vitro* activity against gram-negative, gram-positive aerobic and facultative bacteria including those resistant to cephalosporins, fluoroquinolones, β-lactam/β-lactamase inhibitors, multidrug resistant strains, carbapenem-resistant Enterobacteriaceae, and most anaerobic pathogens.

Limitations

⊕ Not indicated for the treatment of complicated urinary tract infections.

Plazomicin

Aminoglycoside Antibiotic

Approval—June 25, 2018

Indication

- Treatment of complicated UTI infections including pyelonephritis caused by susceptible *E. coli*, *Proteus* and *Enterobacter cloacae*
- Reserved for use in adult patients who have limited or no other treatment options

Mechanism of Action

- Binds to bacterial 30S ribosomal subunit and inhibits protein synthesis.

Pharmacokinetics

- Excretion—renal (90%)
- t½ is 3.5 hours.

Adverse Drug Reactions, Warnings and Precautions

- Hypersensitivity reactions, *Clostridium difficile*-associated diarrhea may occur.
- Impairment of renal function, diarrhea, hypertension, headache, nausea, vomiting and hypotension are other ADRs.

Black Box Warning

Nephrotoxicity, ototoxicity, neuromuscular blockade, fetal toxicity.

Mechanism of Resistance

1. Alteration of the ribosomal target through production of 16S rRNA methyltransferases.
2. Upregulation of efflux pumps.
3. Reduced permeability into bacterial cell due to loss of outer membrane porins.

Drug Interactions

None

Posology

⊕ 15 mg/kg every 24 hours as an IV infusion over 30 minutes for 4 to 7 days.

⊕ Requires dose reduction and therapeutic drug monitoring (plasma trough level <3 µg/mL) in patients with renal impairment.

Advantages

⊕ Not inhibited by most aminoglycosides modifying enzymes (AMEs) known to affect gentamicin, amikacin and tobramycin.

Tafenoquine   Antimalarial

Indication and Approval

1. Radical cure of *Plasmodium vivax* malaria in patients ≥16 years of age (August 8, 2018)
2. Prophylaxis of malaria in >18 years of age (July 20, 2018)

Mechanism of Action

- An 8-aminoquinoline, active against pre-erythrocytic, erythrocytic forms as well as gametocytes of *P. falciparum* and *P. vivax*.
- The exact molecular target of tafenoquine is unknown, but it is postulated that it inhibits hematin polymerization and casues apoptosis like death of the malarial parasite.
- The activity of tafenoquine against the pre-erythrocytic stages of the parasite prevents the development of the erythrocytic forms of the parasite.
- *In vitro*, it also causes red blood cell shrinkage.

Pharmacokinetics

- t½ is 15 days.

Adverse Drug Reactions, Warnings and Precautions

- Headache, dizziness, back pain, diarrhea, nausea, vomiting, increased alanine aminotransferase, insomnia, depression, abnormal dreams, anxiety are common ADRs.
- Hemolytic anemia in G6PD deficiency patients, hypersensitivity reactions and methemoglobinemia may occur.
- Due to a longer t½, psychiatric effects and hypersensitivity reactions may be delayed in onset or prolonged in duration.

Contraindications

In G6PD deficienct individuals:

- During breastfeeding when the infant is found to be G6PD deficient.
- If G6PD status is unknown.
- Known hypersensitivity reaction to the drug
- History of psychotic disorders or current psychotic symptoms

Drug Interactions

Co-administration with substrates of organic cation transporter-2 (OCT2) or multidrug and toxin extrusion (MATE) transporters, should be avoided as their concentrations may increase (e.g. dofetilide, metformin).

Posology

1. *For radical cure:*
   Two 150 mg tablets taken together at once on day 1 and 2 of the antimalarial therapy for the acute *P. vivax* malaria, with food.
2. *For prophylaxis: 200 mg*
   - Loading regimen: OD × 3 days before traveling to an endemic area.
   - Maintenance regimen: Once weekly, start 7 days after last loading dose while in the endemic area.
   - Terminal prophylaxis: 200 mg once 7 days after last maintenance dose.

Advantages

- Long-acting analogue of primaquine; better compliance.

Moxidectin	Anthelmintic

Approval—June 13, 2018

Indication

Treatment of onchocerciasis due to *Onchocerca volvulus* in age >12 years

Mechanism of Action

- Moxidectin is a macrocyclic lactone and a potent endectocide.
- It binds to glutamate-gated chloride channels, GABA receptors and/or ABC transporters of the parasite which mediate the parasite nerve and muscle cell functioning.
- This binding causes an increase in the permeability of the nerve and muscle cells, influx of chloride ions, hyperpolarization of the nerves and flaccid paralysis of the muscles.
- Moxidectin leads to reduction in the
  a. Motility of all stages of the parasite,
  b. Excretion of immunomodulatory proteins,
  c. Fertility of the male and female adult worms.
- Moxidectin is active against the microfilariae of *O. volvulus*.
- Though ineffective in killing the adult worms, moxidectin inhibits intrauterine embryogenesis and release of microfilariae from the adult worms.

Pharmacokinetics

- Minimal hepatic metabolism
- 2% of the dose eliminated unchanged in the feces within the first 72 hours
- Negligilbe renal elimination of intact drug
- t½ is 23 days.

Adverse Drug Reactions, Warnings and Precautions

- Common ADRs are eosinophilia, pruritus, musculoskeletal pain, headache, lymphopenia, tachycardia, rash, abdominal pain, hypotension, pyrexia, leukocytosis, influenza-like illness, neutropenia, cough, lymph node pain, dizziness, diarrhea, hyponatremia, peripheral swelling.

- Mazzotti reaction may occur. Monitor patients for systemic, ocular and dermatological manifestations.
- Encephalopathy in loa loa coinfected patients may occur. Assess patients for loiasis in endemic areas prior to treatment.
- Patients with hyperreactive onchodermatitis (sowda) may experience severe edema and aggravation of onchodermatitis.

Posology

8 mg (four 2 mg tablets) as a single oral dose.

Advantages

- Skin microfilarial loads are lower after moxidectin treatment than after ivermectin suggesting a greater reduction of parasite transmission and accelerating progress towards elimination.

Limitations

- The safety and efficacy of repeat administration is not studied yet.

10 Anticancer Drugs

	Drug	Class	Indication
1.	Apalutamide	Androgen receptor antagonist	Prostate cancer
2.	Abiraterone acetate	CYP17 inhibitor	Prostate cancer
3.	Lutetium Lu177 detonate	Somatostatin analogue	Gastroenteropancreatic neuroendocrine tumors
4.	Ivosidenib	IDH1 inhibitor	Acute myeloid leukemia
5.	Glasdegib	Hedgehog pathway inhibitor	Acute myeloid leukemia
6.	Gilteritinib	FLT3/AXL kinase inhibitor	Acute myeloid leukemia
7.	Calaspargase pegol-mknl	Asparagine specific enzyme (L-asparaginase)	Acute lymphoblastic leukemia
8.	Duvelisib	PI3K-δ and PI3K-γ inhibitor	Chronic lymphocytic leukemia, small lymphocytic lymphoma, follicular lymphoma
9.	Moxetumomab pasudotox-tdfk	CD22 directed cytotoxin	Hairy cell leukemia
10.	Dacomitinib	EGFR inhibitor	Non-small cell lung cancer
11.	Lorlatinib	ALK (anaplastic lymphocyte kinase) inhibitor	Non-small cell lung cancer
12.	Talazoparib	PARP inhibitor	Breast cancer
13.	Cemiplimab–rwlc	PD1 antagonist	Cutaneous squamous cell carcinoma
14.	Mogamulizumab-kpkc	CCR4 antagonist	Mycosis fungoides
15.	Binimetinib	Kinase inhibitor	Metastatic melanoma
16.	Encorafenib	Kinase inhibitor	Metastatic melanoma

17. Iobenguane I-131	Radiopharma-ceutical	Pheochromocytoma, neuroblastoma
18. Larotrectinib	NTRK inhibitor	Solid tumors with NTRK gene fusion
19. Emapalumab-lzsg	IFN-gamma antibody	Primary hemophagocytic lymphohistiocytosis
20 Tagraxofusp-erzs	CD123 directed cytotoxin	Blastic plasmatocytoid dendritic cell neoplasm

Apalutamide
Androgen Receptor Antagonist

Approval—February 14, 2018

Indication

Treatment of non-metastatic castration-resistant prostate cancer

Mechanism of Action

- Apalutamide is an androgen receptor (AR) antagonist which binds to AR's ligand binding domain and inhibits translocation of AR into the nucleus, AR-DNA binding and interferes with AR-mediated transcription, resulting in decreased tumor cell proliferation and increased apoptosis.
- The active metabolite, N-desmethyl apalutamide, has one-third the activity of apalutamide.

Pharmacokinetics

- Peaks at 2 hours
- Steady state at 4 weeks
- Bioavailability is about 100%
- aVd is 276 L
- 96% plasma protein bound
- Metabolized by CYP2C8 and CYP3A4 to form active metabolite, N-desmethyl apalutamide
- Autoinduction occurs, an increase in the clearance is observed over time.
- t½ at steady state is 3 days

Adverse Drug Reactions, Warnings and Precautions

- Common adverse effects are fatigue, hypertension, rash, diarrhea, nausea, weight loss, arthralgia, falls, fractures, hot flushes, anorexia, peripheral edema.
- Hypothyroidism may occur.
- If convulsions occur, do not reintroduce the drug.
- QTc prolongation has been seen with apalutamide and its active metabolite.

Contraindications

Pregnancy

Drug Interactions

Enzyme inducer: Induces CYP3A4, CYP2C19, CYP2C9, UGT, P-gp, BCRP, or OATP1B1. The substrates may lose activity.

Posology

240 mg OD, orally, with or without food along with a GnRH analogue or a previous bilateral orchidectomy.

Advantages

⊕ Improved time to metastasis and metastasis-free survival, as compared to placebo.

Limitations

⊕ Though efficacious, adverse effects are more in the elderly.
⊕ Individuals in the reproductive age have to practice contraception.

Abiraterone Acetate | CYP17 Inhibitor

Approval—May 22, 2018

Indication

Treatment of metastatic castration-resistant androgen sensitive prostate cancer

Mechanism of Action

- Abiraterone acetate is a prodrug and gets converted to Abiraterone by esterases.
- They inhibit 17α-hydroxylase or C17, 20-lyase (CYP17), an androgen biosynthesis enzyme expressed in the testicular, adrenal, and prostatic tumor tissues which catalyzes two sequential reactions:
  1. The conversion of pregnenolone and progesterone to their 17α-hydroxy derivatives by 17α-hydroxylase activity
  2. The subsequent formation of dehydroepiandrosterone (DHEA) and androstenedione, respectively, by C17, 20 lyase activity.

Pharmacokinetics

- Peaks at 2 hours.
- Accumulation occurs.
- Absorption is enhanced with food.
- >99% bound to plasma proteins
- Inactive metabolites are sulfate conjugated and excreted.
- Excretion is via feces.
- t½ is 12 ±5 hours

Adverse Drug Reactions, Warnings and Precautions

- Common ADRs are fatigue, joint swelling or discomfort, edema, hot flushes, diarrhea, vomiting, cough, hypertension, dyspnea, urinary tract infection and contusion.
- Anemia, elevated alkaline phosphatase, hypertriglyceridemia, lymphopenia, hypercholesterolemia, hyperglycemia, elevated serum transaminases, hypophosphatemia, and hypokalemia can occur.

- Caution to be exercised in patients with heart failure: Mineralo-corticoid excess can occur causing hypertension, hypokalemia and fluid retention.
- Monitor for adrenocortical insufficiency. Corticosteroids need to be administered during, before and after stressful conditions.
- Hepatotoxicity necessitates dose reduction or discontinuation; monitoring liver function is advocated.

Contraindications

Partners of women, who are or may become pregnant, category X.

Drug Interactions

Inhibits CYP2D6, avoid co-administration with CYP2D6 substrates having narrow therapeutic index.

Posology

- 1 g, orally, OD with prednisolone 5 mg, orally BD.
- To be taken on empty stomach; no food should be taken for 2 hours before and 1 hour after drug administration, as bioavailability increases with food.
- In moderate hepatic impairment (Child-Pugh Class B), reduce the starting dose to 250 mg OD.
- If a patient develops hepatotoxicity, stop the drug though it may be reintroduced at a lower dose later.

Advantages

- Improved survival and reduced progression is observed, as compared to a placebo.
- No dose modification is needed in those with renal impairment.

Limitations

- Cannot be used in patients with severe hepatic impairment.

Lutetium Lu 177 Detonate

Somatostatin Analogue

Approval—January 26, 2018

Indication

Treatment of somatostatin receptor-positive gastroenteropancreatic neuroendocrine tumors (GEP-NETs) including foregut, midgut, and hindgut neuroendocrine tumors in adults

Mechanism of Action

- A radiolabeled somatostatin analogue that binds to the somatostatin receptors, with highest affinity for subtype 2 (SSRT2).
- On binding to the somatostatin receptor expressing cells, including malignant somatostatin receptor-positive tumors, the drug gets internalized.
- Beta emission from Lu177 induces cellular damage by free radical formation in somatostatin receptor-positive cells and in neighboring cells.

Pharmacokinetics

- aVd is 460 L.
- 43% plasma protein bound
- No hepatic metabolism
- Excreted in urine
- t½ is 71 (±28) hours

Adverse Drug Reactions, Warnings and Precautions

- Common ADRs are lymphopenia, increased GGT (gamma-glutamyl transferase), vomiting, nausea, rise in serum transaminases, hyperglycemia, hypokalemia.
- A risk of radiation exposure exists during and after treatment.
- Myelosuppression, leukemia, and/or secondary myelodysplastic syndrome may occur.
- Frequent urination is advised to prevent renal toxicity.
- Monitor liver function as hepatotoxicity is a complication.
- Risk of infertility exists.

- Neuroendocrine hormonal crisis characterized by flushing, diarrhea, hypotension, bronchoconstriction and/or other features may occur.

Contraindications

Pregnancy; women are advised not to breastfeed.

Drug Interactions

Discontinue long-acting somatostatin analogues for at least 4 weeks and short-acting ones for at least 24 hours prior to each dose.

Posology

- 7.4 GBq (200 mCi) every 8 weeks for a total of 4 doses, intravenously.
- Administer a long-acting octreotide 30 mg IM 4–12 hours after each dose, continue at 4 weekly intervals for 18 months or till disease progression.
- Administer a short-acting octreotide for symptomatic management.
- Premedicate with antiemetics and amino acid solution (to prevent nephrotoxicity).

Ivosidenib

IDH1 Inhibitor

Approval—July 20, 2018

Indication

Treatment of adult patients with relapsed or refractory acute myeloid leukemia (AML) with a susceptible IDH1 mutation

Mechanism of Action

- In leukemia cells, isocitrate dehydrogenase 1 (IDH1) enzyme mutations, R132H and R132C substitutions, lead to an increased level of 2-hydroxyglutarate (2-HG).
- Ivosidenib inhibits the mutant IDH1, at a lower concentration than the wild-type IDH1, causing a decrease in the 2-HG levels and also enhances myeloid differentiation. Reduction in blast counts and increase in percentages of mature myeloid cells occurs.

Pharmacokinetics

- Peaks at 3 hours.
- Steady state at 14 days.
- Food enhances absorption.
- aVd is 234 L.
- Metabolized by CYP3A4.
- Excretion is via feces.
- t½ is 93 hours.

Adverse Drug Reactions, Warnings and Precautions

- Common ADRs are fatigue, leukocytosis, arthralgia, diarrhea, dyspnea, edema, nausea, mucositis, rash, pyrexia, cough, constipation.
- QTc prolongation may occur.
- Discontinue treatment, if the patient develops Guillain-Barré syndrome.
- Noninfectious leukocytosis may develop. Treat with hydroxyurea.

Black Box Warning

Differentiation syndrome, fatal if not treated; initiate corticosteroid therapy and hemodynamic monitoring until symptom resolution. Symptoms are fever, dyspnea, hypoxia, pulmonary infiltrates, pleural or pericardial effusions, rapid weight gain or peripheral edema, hypotension, hepatic, renal, or multiorgan dysfunction.

Contraindications

⊕ Pregnancy and lactation.
⊕ Women are advised to avoid breastfeeding for at least a month after the last dose.

Drug Interactions

⊕ Substrate of CYP3A4, avoid co-administration with inducers or inhibitors.
⊕ Avoid concomitant use with drugs prolonging QTc interval.

Posology

⊕ 500 mg once daily, orally, for a minimum of 6 months, provided there is no disease progression or toxicity.
⊕ Avoid fatty meals.
⊕ Do not take 2 doses within 12 hours.

Advantages

⊕ Complete remissions may occur with 6 months of therapy.

Limitations

⊕ Some patients may remain transfusion dependent.

Glasdegib

Hedgehog Pathway Inhibitor

Approval—November 21, 2018

Indication

In combination with low-dose cytarabine, for the treatment of newly-diagnosed acute myeloid leukemia (AML) in adult patients aged ≥75 years or who have comorbidities that preclude the use of intensive induction chemotherapy

Mechanism of Action

- Glasdegib is a small molecule inhibitor of the hedgehog pathway which binds to and inhibits smoothened, a transmembrane protein involved in hedgehog signal transduction.
- The hedgehog signaling pathway transmits information to embryonic cells required for cell differentiation. Smoothened is a component of the pathway and is encoded by the SMO gene, mutation in which can lead to disproportionate growth of cells.
- The combination with low-dose cytarabine inhibits increase in tumor size and reduces the percentage of CD45 + /CD33 + blasts in the marrow to a greater extent than glasdegib or low-dose cytarabine alone.

Pharmacokinetics

- Absolute bioavailability is 77%.
- Food reduces absorption.
- 91% plasma protein bound.
- aVd is 188 L.
- Metabolized by CYP3A4, CYP2C8, UGT1A9.
- Excreted in urine and feces.
- t½ is 17.4 ±3.7 hours

Adverse Drug Reactions, Warnings and Precautions

- Common ADRs are anemia, fatigue, hemorrhage, febrile neutropenia, musculoskeletal pain, nausea, edema, thrombocytopenia, rash, dyspnea, anorexia, dysgeusia, mucositis, constipation.

- Blood donation must be avoided during and up to 30 days after therapy.
- QTc prolongation can occur.
- Women are advised not to breastfeed.

Black Box Warning

Embryotoxic, fetotoxic, teratogenic. Pregnancy test to be done prior initiation. Contraception is advised for at least 30 days after the last dose.

Contraindications

Pregnancy

Drug Interactions

- Plasma concentration and the risk of QTc prolongation increase when co-administered with CYP3A4 inhibitors.
- Administration with drugs causing QTc prolongation, further increase the risk of QTc prolongation.

Posology

100 mg once daily orally.

Advantages

- Better response, improved survival when given with low-dose cytarabine.

Limitations

- Not studied in patients with severe renal impairment or moderate to severe hepatic impairment.

Gilteritinib

FLT3/AXL Kinase Inhibitor

Approval—November 28, 2018

Indication

Treatment of adult patients who have relapsed or have refractory AML with an FLT3 mutation

Mechanism of Action

A small molecule, Gilteritinib, inhibits multiple receptor tyrosine kinases, including FMS-like tyrosine kinase 3 (FLT3). Gilteritinib also induces apoptosis in leukemic cells expressing FLT3-ITD.

Pharmacokinetics

- Peaks at 4–6 hours.
- Steady state at 15 days.
- Accumulates on repeated dosing.
- Food decreases absorption.
- aVd is 1100 L.
- 94% plasma protein bound.
- Metabolized by CYP3A4.
- Excreted in feces.
- t½ is 113 hours.

Adverse Drug Reactions, Warnings and Precautions

- Common ADRs are myalgia, arthralgia, fatigue, malaise, fever, nausea, vomiting, diarrhea, dyspnea, cough, edema, rash, pneumonia, stomatitis, headache, dizziness, hypotension, raised serum transaminases.
- Posterior reversible encephalopathy syndrome (PRES) may develop. Discontinue the drug.
- Prolongation of QTc interval may be observed. Stop the drug, reintroduce at a lower dose, correct hypokalemia or hypo-magnesemia, if present.
- Stop the drug, if pancreatitis occurs.
- Fetal harm may occur, if administered to a pregnant lady. Contraception is advised.
- Women must not breastfeed.

117

Contraindications

Hypersensitivity to the drug or excipients

Drug Interactions

- *P-gp substrate:* Plasma concentration falls when given with an inducer.
- *CYP3A4 substrate:* Avoid co-administration with strong inducers or inhibitors.

Posology

- 120 mg OD, orally.
- Alteration is not needed in mild to moderate hepatic or renal impairment.

Advantages

- Response is seen as early as 0.9 months.
- Reduced need for transfusions was observed, both during the clinical trials and the follow-up period.

Calaspargase Pegol-mknl

Asparagine Specific Enzyme

Approval—December 20, 2018

Indication

Treatment of acute lymphoblastic leukemia in patients aged 1 month to 21 years as a part of multidrug chemotherapy

Mechanism of Action

- The drug is an asparagine-specific enzyme (L-asparaginase).
- L-asparaginase aids the conversion of L-asparagine to aspartic acid and ammonia.
- Leukemic cells require L-asparagine for survival.
- The drug specifically targets leukemic cells which lack or have reduced asparagine synthetase and depend on exogenous L-asparagine for survival.

Pharmacokinetics

t½ is 16.1 days.

Adverse Drug Reactions, Warnings and Precautions

- Common ADRs are elevated serum transaminases and/or bilirubin, pancreatitis, prolongation of aPTT, decreased blood fibrinogen levels.
- Fungal infections, pneumonia, arrhythmias and cardiac failure are infrequent.
- Hypersensitivity reactions, pancreatitis, hepatotoxicity, thrombosis and/or hemorrhage may occur.
- Potential fetal harm may occur, if administered to a pregnant lady. Non-oral contraception is advised for at least 3 months after the last dose.
- Women must not breastfeed for at least 3 months after the last dose.

Contraindications

- Hypersensitivity to the active ingredient or any of the components

- History of thrombosis or hemorrhagic events with L-asparaginase therapy
- History of pancreatitis with L-asparaginase therapy
- Severe hepatic impairment

Drug Interactions

The efficacy of estrogen and progesterone reduces when co-administered with calaspargase pegol-mknl.

Posology

2500 units/m^2 IV every 21 days.

Advantages

- Less frequent administration as compared to pegaspargase to achieve the same serum asparaginase activity with similar toxicity.

Duvelisib   PI3K-δ & PI3K-γ Inhibitor

Approval—September 24, 2018

Indications

- Relapsed or refractory chronic lymphocytic leukemia (CLL) or small lymphocytic lymphoma (SLL) after at least two prior therapies
- Relapsed or refractory follicular lymphoma (FL) after at least two prior systemic therapies

Mechanism of Action

- Duvelisib is a dual inhibitor of phosphatidylinositol 3 kinases, PI3K-δ and PI3K-γ, expressed in normal and malignant cells.
- It causes inhibition of growth as well as reduces the viability of the cell lines derived from malignant B cells and primary CLL tumor cells.
- Other mechanisms, by which Duvelisib acts, include:
  - B cell receptor signaling
  - CXCR12-mediated chemotaxis of malignant B cells
  - CXCL12-induced T cell migration
  - M-CSF and IL-4 driven M2 polarization of macrophages

Pharmacokinetics

- Peaks at 1 to 2 hours.
- Absolute bioavailability is 42%.
- Food reduces absorption.
- 98% plasma protein bound.
- aVd is 28.5 L.
- Metabolized by CYP3A4.
- Excreted in feces.
- $t\frac{1}{2}$ is 4.7 hours.

Adverse Drug Reactions, Warnings and Precautions

- Common ADRs are diarrhea or colitis, neutropenia, rash, fatigue, pyrexia, cough, nausea, upper respiratory tract infection, pneumonia, musculoskeletal pain, and anemia.

- Hepatotoxicity, neutropenia, thrombocytopenia may occur.
- Embryo-fetal toxicity may occur. Contraception is advised for at least 1 month after the last dose. Women are advised no to breastfeed.

Black Box Warning

Fatal and/or serious infections, diarrhea, cutaneous reactions, pneumonitis may occur. Withhold the drug.

Contraindications

None

Drug Interactions

- CYP3A substrate and inhibitor. Adjust dose when co-administered with CYP3A inducers, inhibitors or substrates.
- In vitro, substrate of P-gp and BCRP.

Posology

- 25 mg BD, orally.

Advantages

- Slower progression, prolonged survival, better overall response in patients of CLL or SLL as compared to ofatumumab.
- A good response is seen in those with follicular lymphoma as well.

Moxetumomab Pasudotox-tdfk

CD22-directed Cytotoxin

Approval—September 13, 2018

Indication

Treatment of adult patients with relapsed or refractory hairy cell leukemia (HCL) who have received at least two prior systemic therapies, including treatment with a purine nucleoside analog (PNA)

Mechanism of Action

A recombinant murine immunoglobulin directed to CD22, moxetumomab pasudotox-tdfk, binds to CD22 on the surface of B cells and gets internalized where the complex inhibits ADP-ribosylation of elongation factor 2, protein synthesis and causes apoptotic cell death.

Pharmacokinetics

- Does not accumulate.
- aVd is 6.5 L.
- Metabolized proteolytically.
- t½ is 1.4 hours.

Adverse Drug Reactions, Warnings and Precautions

- Common ADRs are infusion related reactions, edema, nausea, fatigue, headache, pyrexia, constipation, anemia, and diarrhea.
- Rise in serum creatinine/ALT/AST, hypoalbuminemia, hypocalcemia, hypophosphatemia may occur.
- Renal toxicity is a possibility. Withhold treatment till recovery.
- Electrolyte abnormalities can occur. Monitor and replace.
- Contraception is recommended till at least 1 month after the last dose.
- Women are advised not to breastfeed.

Black Box Warning

- *Life-threatening capillary leak syndrome (CLS):* Delaying dosing or discontinuation is recommended.
- *Life-threatening hemolytic uremic syndrome (HUS):* Discontinue therapy.

Contraindications

None

Drug Interactions

None

Posology

- 0.04 mg/kg IV infusion over 30 minutes on days 1, 3, 5 of each 28-day cycle.
- Maintaining hydration with 1L NS over 2–4 hours after each infusion and 2–3 L of oral fluid per day for days 1 to 8 of every cycle is to be advised to all patients.
- Administer low dose aspirin on days 1 to 8 of each 28-day cycle as thromboprophylaxis.
- Premedicate with an antipyretic, antihistamine, H_2 receptor antagonist prior to all infusions.
- Post-medication management with antihistamines, antipyretics and corticosteroids may be needed.
- No dose changes are needed in those with mild hepatic or renal impairment.

Limitations

- Antibody to the drug may develop, reducing its bioavailability.
- Cannot be used in patients with severe renal impairment.
- Adverse effects leading to discontinuation are more amongst the elderly.

Dacomitinib

EGFR Inhibitor

Approval—September 27, 2018

Indication

Treatment of patients with metastatic non-small cell lung cancer (NSCLC) with epidermal growth factor receptor (EGFR) exon 19 deletion or exon 21 L858R substitution mutations

Mechanism of Action

Dacomitinib inhibits the kinase activity of EGFR family (EGFR/HER1, HER2, and HER4 and certain EGFR activating mutations like exon 19 deletion or the exon 21 L858R substitution mutation) irreversibly. It also causes a dose-dependent inhibition of EGFR and HER2 autophosphorylation and tumor growth.

Pharmacokinetics

- Peaks at 6 hours.
- Steady state at 14 days.
- Oral bioavailability is 80%.
- aVd is 1889 L.
- Metabolized by CYP2D6 to form active metabolite O-desmethyl dacomitinib (in vitro) and CYP3A4 into minor metabolites.
- Excreted in feces.
- t½ is 70 hours.

Adverse Drug Reactions, Warnings and Precautions

- Common ADRs are diarrhea, rash, paronychia, stomatitis, decreased appetite, dry skin, weight loss, alopecia, cough, pruritus.
- Interstitial lung disease may occur requiring permanent discontinuation of the drug.
- Withhold and reduce dose, if diarrhea or severe dermatological reactions occur.
- Embryo-fetal toxicity may occur. Contraception is advised till at least 17 days after the last dose.
- Women are advised not to breastfeed.

Contraindications

None

Drug Interactions

⊕ Avoid co-administration of proton pump inhibitors. Locally acting antacids or H_2 blockers can be used. However, dacomitinib should not be administered for at least 6 hours before to 10 hours after H_2 blockers.

⊕ CYP2D6 inhibitor: May increase the plasma concentration of the substrate.

Posology

⊕ 45 mg once daily, orally.

⊕ Higher doses lead to toxicity.

⊕ No adjustment is required in those with mild to moderate hepatic or renal impairment.

Advantages

⊕ Median progression free survival as well as duration of response are significantly better as compared to gefitinib.

Limitations

⊕ The overall response rate was similar with dacomitinib and gefitinib.

Lorlatinib

ALK Inhibitor

Approval—November 2, 2018

Indication

Adult patients with anaplastic lymphoma kinase (ALK)-positive metastatic NSCLC whose disease has progressed on:
- Crizotinib and at least one other ALK inhibitor for metastatic disease; or
- Alectinib as the first ALK inhibitor therapy for metastatic disease; or
- Ceritinib as the first ALK inhibitor therapy for metastatic disease

Mechanism of Action

- Lorlatinib is a kinase inhibitor with *in vitro* activity against ALK and ROS1 as well as TYK1, FER, FPS, TRKA, TRKB, TRKC, FAK, FAK2, and ACK and some mutant forms of ALK enzyme.
- Anti-tumor activity is observed in mice with implanted tumors comprising of EML4 fusions with either ALK variant 1 or ALK mutations, including the G1202R and I1171T mutations.

Pharmacokinetics

- Peaks at 1.2 hours.
- Absolute bioavailability is 81%.
- aVd is 305 L.
- 66% plasma protein bound.
- Metabolized by CYP3A4, UGT1A4, with minor contribution from CYP2C8/2C19/3A5 and UGT1A3.
- t½ is 24 hours.

Adverse Drug Reactions, Warnings and Precautions

- Common ADRs are edema, peripheral neuropathy, fatigue, dyspnea, diarrhea, weight gain, arthralgia.
- CNS effects: Seizures, hallucinations, changes in cognitive function, mood (including suicidal ideation), speech, mental status, and sleep. Stop and reintroduce or permanently discontinue, as appropriate.

- Hyperlipidemia: Lipid lowering drugs should be co-administered.
- AV block, interstitial lung disease, pneumonitis are potential complications. Stop and reintroduce, reduce the dose or permanently discontinue, as appropriate.
- Embryo-fetal toxicity can occur. Contraception, non-hormonal, is advised for at least 6 months in females and 3 months in males, after the last dose.
- Women are advised not to breastfeed.

Contraindications

With strong CYP3A4 inducers: Serious hepatotoxicity. The inducers should be discontinued for at least 3 half-lives of the drug prior to its administration.

Drug Interactions

CYP3A substrate and inducer, drug interactions can occur.

Posology

100 mg once daily, orally.

Talazoparib

PARP Inhibitor

Approval—October 16, 2018

Indication

Individuals with deleterious or suspected deleterious germline BRCA-mutated (gBRCAm) HER2-negative locally advanced or metastatic breast cancer

Mechanism of Action

- Talazoparib is a poly ADP ribose polymerase (PARP) inhibitor, inhibits both PARP1 and PARP2, which play a role in DNA repair.
- Inhibition of PARP enzymatic activity leads to an increase in the formation of PARP-DNA complexes resulting in DNA damage, decreased cell proliferation, and apoptosis and is seen specifically in those with BRCA mutations.

Pharmacokinetics

- Peaks at 1 to 2 hours.
- Food decreases absorption.
- aVd is 420 L.
- Plasma protein binding, 74%.
- Metabolized minimally in the liver.
- Excreted in urine.
- t½ is 90 ±58 hours.

Adverse Drug Reactions, Warnings and Precautions

- Common ADRs are fatigue, anemia, neutropenia, thrombo-cytopenia, nausea, vomiting, diarrhea, anorexia, hypocalcemia, raised serum transaminases, alopecia, headache.
- Myelosuppression, myelodysplastic syndrome or AML may occur.
- Embryofetal toxicity can occur. Contraception must be employed.

Contraindications

Pregnancy, lactation

Drug Interactions

- P-gp substrate, dose reduction is needed, if co-administered with a P-gp inhibitor.
- BCRP substrate, dose reduction is needed, if co-administered with a BCRP inhibitor.

Posology

- 1 mg once daily, orally.
- Renal impairment (moderate, CLcr 30–59 mL/min)—0.75 mg OD, orally.

Advantages

- No dose changes are required in the elderly.

Limitations

- Safety in moderate to severe hepatic impairment is not known.

Cemiplimab-rwlc

PD-1 Antagonist

Approval—September 28, 2018

Indication

Metastatic cutaneous squamous cell carcinoma (CSCC) or locally advanced CSCC who are not candidates for curative surgery or curative radiation

Mechanism of Action

- Cemiplimab-rwlc is a recombinant human programmed death receptor-1 (PD-1) blocking IgG4 antibody which binds to PD-1 and blocks its interaction with PD-L1 and PD-L2.
- Binding of the PD-1 ligands, PD-L1 and PD-L2, to the PD-1 receptor expressed on T cells, inhibits T cell proliferation and cytokine production.
- Upregulation of PD-1 ligands occurs in some tumors and contributes to the inhibition of active T cell immune surveillance of tumors which is inhibited by Cemiplimab-rwlc.

Pharmacokinetics

- t½ is 19 days.

Adverse Drug Reactions, Warnings and Precautions

- Fatigue, rash and diarrhea are common.
- Severe and fatal immune-mediated adverse reactions can occur in any organ system or tissue, including immune-mediated pneumonitis, colitis, hepatitis, endocrinopathies, dermatologic adverse reactions or nephritis and renal dysfunction. Monitor, withhold or permanently discontinue the drug, administer corticosteroids depending on the severity of the reaction.
- In case of infusion reactions, interrupt, slow the rate of infusion or permanently discontinue the drug.
- Embryo-fetal toxicity can occur. Contraception is advised for at least 4 months after the last dose.
- Women are advised not to breastfeed.

Contraindications

None

Posology

350 mg as IV infusion over 30 minutes every 3 weeks.
No changes needed in mild renal/hepatic impairment.

Advantages

⊕ A good partial response is seen in almost 50% patients in metastatic, locally advanced or combined CSCC.

Mogamulizumab-kpkc   CCR4 Antagonist

Approval—August 8, 2018

Indication

Treatment of adult patients with relapsed or refractory mycosis fungoides or Sézary syndrome after at least one prior systemic therapy

Mechanism of action

- Mogamulizumab-kpkc is a defucosylated, humanized IgG1 kappa monoclonal which inhibits CCR4-mediated T cell depletion.
- It binds to CCR4, a G protein-coupled receptor for chemokines involved in the trafficking of lymphocytes to various organs, which target the cell for antibody-dependent cellular cytotoxicity (ADCC) resulting in their depletion.
- CCR4 is expressed on the surface of some T cell malignancies, regulatory T cells (Treg) and a subset of Th2 T cells.

Pharmacokinetics

- $t\frac{1}{2}$ is 17 days.

Adverse Drug Reactions, Warnings and Precautions

- Common ADRs are rash, infusion related reactions, fatigue, diarrhea, musculoskeletal pain, URTI.
- Temporary or permanent discontinuation of the drug is recommended for severe dermatologic, infusion reactions.
- Monitoring and prompt treatment is a must, if infections occur.
- Autoimmune complications may require interruption or permanent discontinuation, as appropriate.
- Complications of allogeneic HSCT may occur. Monitor for severe acute graft-versus-host disease (GVHD) and steroid-refractory GVHD. Transplant-related mortality can occur.
- Contraception is advised for at least 3 months after the last dose.

Contraindications

None

Posology

- 1 mg/kg as IV infusion over at least 60 minutes on days 1, 8, 15, and 22 of the first 28-day cycle and on days 1 and 15 of each subsequent cycle.
- If an infusion reaction occurs, premedication is to be administered for subsequent doses.
- Dose changes are not required in renal impairment and mild-to-moderate hepatic impairment.

Advantages

- Improved survival is seen as compared to Vorinostat.

Limitations

- Hepatitis B reactivation and stress cardiomyopathy may occur.

Binimetinib

Kinase Inhibitor

Approval—June 7, 2018

Indication

In combination with encorafenib, for the treatment of patients with unresectable or metastatic melanoma with BRAF V600E or V600K mutation

Mechanism of Action

- Binimetinib is a reversible inhibitor of mitogen-activated extracellular signal regulated kinase 1 (MEK1) and MEK2 activity.
- MEK proteins are upstream regulators of the extracellular signal-related kinase (ERK) pathway.
- Binimetinib and encorafenib target two different kinases in the RAS/RAF/MEK/ERK pathway and inhibit proliferative activity of BRAF mutation-positive cell lines, especially the ones with BRAF V600E mutation.

Pharmacokinetics

- 50% absorbed orally
- 97% plasma protein bound
- aVd is 92 L.
- Metabolized by UGT1A1 (major) as well as CYP1A2 and CYP2C19 to produce the active metabolite M3
- Excreted in feces (major) and urine.
- t½ is 3.5 hours.

Adverse Drug Reactions, Warnings and Precautions

- Most common ADRs, in combination with encorafenib, are fatigue, nausea, diarrhea, vomiting, and abdominal pain.
- Cardiomyopathy: Assessment of left ventricular ejection fraction before and 2–3 months after therapy.
- Ocular toxicities like retinopathy, retinal vein occlusion and uveitis warrant regular ophthalmological examination.
- DVT, pulmonary embolism, interstitial lung disease, hepatotoxicity, hemorrhage, rhabdomyolysis: Monitoring and prompt treatment is recommended.

⊕ Contraception up to at least 30 days after the last dose is advised. Women are advised not to breastfeed.

Contraindications

None

Posology

⊕ 45 mg twice daily, orally, with encorafenib.

⊕ 30 mg twice daily, orally, in those with moderate-to-severe hepatic impairment.

Advantages

⊕ As compared to vemurafenib, significant improvement in the progression free survival is observed.

Limitations

⊕ Frequent monitoring is a must due to the possibility of various side effects.

Encorafenib   Kinase Inhibitor

Approval—June 27, 2018

Indication

In combination with binimetinib, for the treatment of patients with unresectable or metastatic melanoma with a BRAF V600E or V600K mutation

Mechanism of Action

- Mutation in the BRAF gene leads to constitutive activation of the kinases which in turn stimulate tumor cell growth.
- Encorafenib is a kinase inhibitor. It targets BRAF V600E, as well as wild-type BRAF and CRAF in *in vitro* cell-free assays and induces tumor regression which are associated with RAF/MEK/ERK pathway suppression.

Pharmacokinetics

- Peaks at 2 hours.
- Steady state at 15 days.
- Fatty food reduces absorption.
- 86% plasma protein bound.
- Metabolized by CYP3A4 (major), CYP2C19 and CYP2D6
- Excreted in urine and feces.
- t½ is 3.5 hours.

Adverse Drug Reactions, Warnings and Precautions

- ADRs with binimetinib: Fatigue, nausea, vomiting, abdominal pain, arthralgia.
- New primary malignancies, cutaneous and non-cutaneous, may occur. Monitoring is a must.
- Proliferation of BRAF wild-type tumors may occur with BRAF inhibitors.
- Hemorrhage, uveitis, QTc prolongation warrant monitoring.
- Embryo-fetal toxicity warrants the use of contraceptives, non-hormonal, for at least 2 weeks after the last dose. Women are advised not to breastfeed.

Contraindications

None

Drug Interactions

⊕ Substrate and inhibitor of CYP3A4.
⊕ Coadministration with CYP3A4 inducers, inhibitors or substrates warrants dose modification.

Posology

450 mg once daily, orally, in combination with binimetinib.

Advantages

⊕ The combination provides a longer progression free survival with a better overall response rate as compared to vemurafenib.

Limitations

⊕ Not indicated for treatment of patients with wild-type BRAF melanoma.
⊕ May impair fertility in males.

Iobenguane I-131   Radiopharmaceutical

Approval—July 20, 2018

Indication

Detection of primary or metastatic pheochromocytoma or neuroblastoma as an adjunct to other diagnostic tests

Mechanism of Action

- Iobenguane is structurally similar to guanethidine and norepinephrine.
- It is taken up by the NE transporters at the adrenergic nerve endings and is stored pre-synaptic vesicles and gets accumulated in the adrenal medulla, salivary glands, heart, liver, spleen and lungs as well as tumors derived from the neural crest.
- Radiolabeling makes obtaining scintigraphic images of the tissues where the drug accumulates possible.
- It aids easy visualization of adrenergic tissues.

Pharmacokinetics

- Rapidly cleared form blood.
- Accumulates in the adrenergically innervated tissues.
- Excreted in the urine, 90% within 4 days.
- Not cleared by dialysis.

Adverse Drug Reactions, Warnings and Precautions

- Common ADRs are dizziness, rash, pruritus, flushing and injection site hemorrhage.
- Serious hypersensitivity reactions can occur.
- It contains benzyl alcohol which may cause serious reactions in premature or low birth weight infants.
- Greater radiation exposure occurs in those with severe renal impairment.
- If pre-treatment with anti-thyroid drugs is not done, I^{131} accumulates in the thyroid gland.
- Monitoring of blood pressure before and 30 minutes after iobenguane administration is required as hypertension can occur.

Contraindications

- Known hypersensitivity to iobenguane or iobenguane sulfate
- Pregnant, lactating women
- Children <1 month, as efficacy has not been established

Drug Interactions

Drugs which inhibit NET, deplete NE stores or inhibit its reuptake, sympathomimetic amines and cocaine, decrease the uptake of iobenguane in the neuroendocrine tumors. Their administration should be withheld for 5 half-lives prior to iobeguane administration.

Posology

- Pre-treat with anti-thyroid drugs.
- For patients ≥16 years or <16 years of age and ≥70 kg: 10 mCi (370 MBq).
- For patients <16 years of age and <70 kg: Scaled to the adult reference activity based on weight.
- Administered IV over 1–2 minutes followed by an injection of NS to ensure full delivery of iobenguane.

Larotrectinib   NTRK Inhibitor

Approval—November 26, 2018

Indication

Treatment of adult and pediatric patients with solid tumors that:
- have a neurotrophic receptor tyrosine kinase (NTRK) gene fusion without a known acquired resistance mutation,
- are metastatic or where surgical resection is likely to result in severe morbidity, and
- have no satisfactory alternative treatments or that have progressed following treatment.

Mechanism of Action

- Larotrectinib is an inhibitor of the tropomyosin receptor kinases (TRK), TRKA, TRKB, and TRKC.
- TRKA, B, and C are encoded by the genes NTRK1, NTRK2, and NTRK3. Chromosomal rearrangements involving these genes result in constitutively activated chimeric TRK fusion proteins that act as an oncogenic drivers, promoting cell proliferation and survival in tumor cell lines which is inhibited by larotrectinib.

Pharmacokinetics

- Absolute bioavailability is 34%.
- Fatty food reduces absorption.
- aVd is 48 L.
- 70% bound to plasma proteins.
- Metabolized by CYP3A4.
- Excreted in urine and feces.
- t½ is 2.9 hours.

Adverse Drug Reactions, Warnings and Precautions

- Common ADRs are fatigue, nausea, dizziness, vomiting, raised transaminases, cough, constipation, diarrhea.
- Neurotoxicity may occur.
- Contraception is advised till at least 1 week after the last dose. Women are advised not to breastfeed.

Contraindications

Pregnancy

Drug Interactions

Larotrectinib is a CYP3A4 substrate and inhibitor, dose adjustment is required when co-administered with other CYP3A4 substrates, inducers and inhibitors.

Posology

- BSA ≥ 1.0 m^2: 100 mg BD, orally.
- BSA < 1.0 m^2: 100 mg/m^2 BD, orally.
- Dose reduction is recommended in those with moderate to severe hepatic failure.

Advantages

- Overall response rate of 75% in those with solid tumors with 63% responding even after 9 months of therapy.

Emapalumab-lzsg   IFN-gamma Antibody

Approval—November 20, 2018

Indication

Treatment of adult and pediatric patients with primary hemophagocytic lymphohistiocytosis (HLH) having refractory, recurrent or progressive disease or intolerance with conventional HLH therapy

Mechanism of Action

- A raised level of interferon gamma (IFNγ) is seen in patients of HLH, indicating a possible role of IFNγ in the pathogenesis of HLH.
- Emapalumab-lzsg is a monoclonal antibody which binds to and neutralizes IFNγ.

Pharmacokinetics

- t½ in healthy individuals is 22 days while in those with HLH may vary from 2.5 to 18.9 days.

Adverse Drug Reactions, Warnings and Precautions

- Common ADRs are infections, hypertension, infusion-related reactions, fever.
- Prophylaxis for herpes zoster, *Pneumocystis jirovecii* and fungal infections may be required.
- Live vaccines should not be co-administered.
- Infusion should be interrupted, if the infusion reactions are severe.

Contraindications

None

Drug Interactions

The formation of CYP450 enzymes may be suppressed by increased levels of IFNγ during chronic inflammation. By neutralizing IFNγ, Emapalumab may normalize CYP450 activities which may reduce the efficacy of drugs that are CYP450 substrates due to increased

143

metabolism. Upon initiation or discontinuation of the drug, monitor for reduced efficacy and adjust dosage of CYP450 substrates as appropriate.

Posology

- 1 mg/kg as an IV infusion over 1 hour twice a week.
- Prednisolone to be administered concomitantly.

Advantages

- A good overall response and an improved survival has been reported with emapalumab-lzsg.

Limitations

- Little is known about the pharmacokinetics and drug-drug interactions.

Tagraxofusp-erzs

CD123-Directed Cytotoxin

Approval—December 21, 2018

Indication

Treatment of blastic plasmacytoid dendritic cell neoplasm (BPDCN) in patients aged >2 years

Mechanism of Action

- BPDCN is a rare form of hematological malignancy of the plasmacytoid dendritic cells.
- Malignant cells overexpress CD123 which is IL-3 receptor and is required for their survival.
- Tagraxofusp-erzs is CD123-directed cytotoxin. It is a fusion protein of recombinant human interleukin-3 (IL-3) and truncated diphtheria toxin (DT).
- It binds to CD123 and gets internalized to release the diphtheria toxin. The toxin then binds to the ADP-ribosylation elongation factor 2 which plays a role in protein translation. Tagraxofusp-erzs thus inhibits protein synthesis and causes apoptosis in CD123 expressing cells.

Pharmacokinetics

- aVd is 5.1L.
- t½ is 0.7 hours (51 minutes)
- Antidrug antibodies in the plasma and reduced free drug concentration in the plasma are observed.

Adverse Drug Reactions, Warnings and Precautions

- Common ADRs are capillary leak syndrome, nausea, fatigue, peripheral edema, hypertension, pyrexia, weight gain.
- Laboratory abnormalities: Decrease in albumin, platelets, hemoglobin, calcium, sodium; increase in glucose and serum transaminases.
- Hypersensitivity reactions and hepatotoxicity may occur.
- Women are advised not to breastfeed 1 week after the last dose.
- There is a potential risk to the fetus, if administered in a pregnant woman. Contraception is advised for at least 1 week after the last dose.

145

Black Box Warning

Capillary leak syndrome (CLS), which may be life-threatening or fatal if not adequately managed, can occur.

Contraindications

None

Posology

- Pretreat with H_1 and H_2 receptor antagonists, acetaminophem and corticosteroids.
- Administer tagraxofusp-erzs IV at 12 µg/kg over 15 minutes, once daily on days 1 through 5 of the 21-day cycle.
- First cycle to be administered in in-patient setting.

Advantages

- First in class for treatment of BPCDN.
- It acts as an alternative to intensive chemotherapy followed by bone marrow transplantation.
- Complete remission is seen in 50% of treatment naïve individuals.
- Response occur as early as 3.9 months but may be delayed up to 12.2 months.
- Holds an orphan drug status.
- Classified as breakthrough therapy.

Limitations

- Complete remission in relapse and refractory cases is not very impressive.

1. Danoprevir: 8th June 2018, China

- NS3 protease inhibitor.
- *Indication:* In combination with ritonavir, peg-interferon alfa and ribavirin for use in treatment-naive, non-cirrhotic, chronic hepatitis C genotype 1b-infected adult patients
- *Mechanism of action:* It forms an initial collision complex with NS3 protease of Hepatitis C virus which subsequently isomerizes to a highly stable complex from which danoprevir dissociates slowly, thereby inhibiting viral replication.
- Danoprevir is a substrate of CYP3A. Its coadminstration with ritonavir; a CYP3A inhibitor enhances the exposure to danoprevir and can be used to reduce the dose of danoprevir while improving tolerability and maintaining efficacy.
- *Adverse events:* Anemia, fever, fatigue, headache, influenza-like symptoms, dizziness, anorexia, rash, diarrhea.
- *Dose:* 100 mg twice daily administered in combination with ritonavir, peg-interferon alfa-2a.

2. Caplacizumab: 3rd September 2018, Europe

- Humanized single-variable domain immunoglobulin (nanobody)
- *Indication:* Treatment of acquired thrombotic thrombo-cytopenic purpura (aTTP) in adults in conjunction with plasma exchange and immunosuppression
- *Mechanism of action:* Targets the A1-domain of the von Willebrand factor and inhibits the interaction between von Willebrand factor and platelets, thus preventing platelet adhesion.
- *Adverse events:* Gingival bleeding, epistaxis, headache, fatigue, urticarial, injection site reactions.
- *Dose:*
  - 10 mg IV prior to plasma exchange.
  - 10 mg SC daily after completion of each plasma exchange till the time the patient is receiving daily plasma exchange treatment.
  - 10 mg SC injection daily × 30 days after stopping daily plasma exchange treatment.

- In case the immunological disease remains unresolved at the end of the above regimen, it is advised to optimize the immunosuppression regimen and continue daily SC injections of Caplacizumab 10 mg until the signs of underlying immunological disease are resolved.

3. Pyrotinib: August 2018, China
- Tyrosine kinase inhibitor
- *Indication:* In combination with Capecitabine for the treatment of HER2 positive advanced or metastatic breast cancer in patients previously treated with anthracycline or taxane chemotherapy.
- *Mechanism of action*
  - Irreversible tyrosine kinase inhibitor with activity against EGFR/HER1, HER2 and HER4.
  - Inhibits HER2 factor-directed tumor growth and HER2-mediated downstream signaling.
  - Blocks the tumor cells in the G1 phase of the cell cycle.
- *Pharmacokinetics:* t½ is 18.2 hours, metabolized by CYP3A4, mainly excreted in feces.
- *Adverse events:* Nausea, vomiting, diarrhea, hand and foot syndrome, leukopenia, and neutropenia.
- *Dose:* 400 mg oral once daily after a meal.

4. Fruquintinib: 4th September 2018, China
- VEGFR inhibitor
- *Indication:* Treatment of metastatic colorectal cancer in patients who have failed at least two prior systemic antineoplastic therapies, including fluoropyrimidine, oxaliplatin and irinotecan, with or without prior use of anti-VEGF or anti-epidermal growth factor receptor (EGFR) therapies.
- *Mechanism of action:* Potent, highly selective small molecule inhibitor of VEGFR-1, 2 and 3.
- *Pharmacokinetics:* t½ is 42 hours, extensively metabolized and excreted in urine (60%) and feces (30%).
- *Adverse events:* Hypertension, hand-foot skin reaction, proteinuria, dysphonia, TSH elevation.
- *Dose:* 5 mg oral once daily for 21 days followed by a break of 7 days in every 28-day cycle.

5. Vibegron: September 2018, Japan
- Beta 3 adrenergic receptor agonist.

- *Indication:* Treatment of urgency, urinary frequency, urge incontinence and urinary incontinence in overactive bladder
- *Mechanism of action:* Beta-3 adrenoreceptors are predominantly expressed in human bladder tissue. Beta-3 agonist causes smooth muscle relaxation in the bladder to increase the bladder capacity.
- *Pharmacokinetics:* t½ is 60–70 hours, predominantly excreted unchanged in feces.
- *Plasma drug interactions* concentrations may increase when co-administered with drugs that inhibit CYP3A4 and P-gp and reduce when co-administered with drugs that induce CYP3A4 and P-gp.
- *Dose:* 50 mg orally once daily after food. Dose adjustments are required when administered to the elderly or those with severe liver dysfunction.
- *Advantages:* Anticholinergic therapy currently used for overactive bladder has notable problems like low adherence rate, inadequate effectiveness and adverse drug reactions such as dry mouth, constipation and cognitive impairment. Therefore, selective beta-3 adrenergic therapy is a novel, potent, alternative therapy with excellent pharmacological activity.

6. Omidenepag isopropyl: September 2018, Japan

- Selective prostaglandin E2 receptor 2 (EP2) agonist with a non-prostaglandin structure.
- *Indication:* Treatment of glaucoma and ocular hypertension
- *Mechanism of action:* Increases the uveoscleral and the trabecular outflow of aqueous humor causing reduction in intraocular pressure (IOP).
- *Pharmacokinetics:* t½ is 0.5 hour.
- *Warning and precautions:* It may worsen eye inflammation in patients with ocular inflammatory diseases such as iritis, uveitis and cystoid macular edema.
- *Adverse drug reactions:* Conjunctival hyperemia, macular edema (occasional).
- *Dose:* 1 drop of 0.002% ophthalmic solution in the eye, once daily.

Appendix 2: New Formulations of Existing Drugs

	Drug	Formulation	Indication
	Drug	*Formulation*	*Indication*
	Central Nervous System		
1	Amantadine hydrochloride	Extended release tablet	Parkinson's disease; Extrapyramidal reactions
2	Levodopa	Inhalation powder	Parkinson's disease
3	Buprenorphine-naloxone	Sublingual film	Opioid dependence–maintenance
4	Clobazam	Oral film	Lennox-Gastaut syndrome
5	Desmopressin acetate	Sublingual tablet	Nocturia
6	Lidocaine	Transdermal patch	Postherpetic neuralgia
7	Methyl-phenidate hydrochloride	Extended release capsules	Attention deficit hyperactivity disorder (ADHD)
8	Riluzole	Oral suspension	Amyotrophic lateral sclerosis
9	Risperidone	Extended release injectable suspension	Schizophrenia
10	Sufentanil	Sublingual tablet	Pain
	Cardiovascular System		
11	Levoleucovorin	Intravenous injection	Folic acid antagonist overdose
	Respiratory System		
12	Epinephrine	Inhalation aerosol, mist	Asthma
13	Albuterol sulfate	Inhalation powder	Bronchospasm prophylaxis, asthma, COPD
	Endocrine System		
14	Testosterone enanthate	Subcutaneous injection	Male hypogonadism
15	Estradiol	Vaginal insert	Dyspareunia
	Ophthalmology		
16	Cyclosporine	Ophthalmic solution	Keratoconjunctivitis sicca
17	Dexamethasone	Intraocular suspension	Postoperative ocular inflammation
18	Dexamethasone	Ophthalmic insert	Postoperative ocular inflammation
19	Fluocinolone acetonide	Intravitreal implant	Non-infectious posterior segment uveitis

Contd...

20	Latanoprost	Ophthalmic emulsion	Open angle hlaucoma; intraocular hypertension
Antimicrobial agents			
21	Vancomycin hydrochloride	Oral solution	*Clostridium difficile*-associated diarrhea; enterocolitis
22	Rifamycin	Delayed release tablets	Traveler's diarrhea
23	Itraconazole	Capsule	Blastomycosis, histoplasmosis, aspergillosis
Dermatology			
24	Glycopyrronium	Cloth	Primary axillary hyperhidrosis
25	Tretinoin	0.05% lotion	Acne
26	Halobetasol proprionate	Lotion	Plaque psoriasis
Cancer chemotherapy			
27	Levoleucovorin	Intravenous injection	Methotrexate toxicity colorectal cancer
Gastroenterology			
28	Prucalopride	Initially approved in Europe, now approved by the US-FDA	Chronic idiopathic constipation

Appendix 3: New Fixed Dose Combinations with Old Drugs

	Drugs	Indication
1	Amlodipine-celecoxib	Hypertension with osteoarthritis
2	Acetaminophen-benzhydrocodone	Severe acute pain
3	Ethinyl estradiol, levonorgestrel, ferrous bisglycinate (as a placebo)	Oral contraceptive
4	Doravirine, lamivudine, tenofovir disoproxil fumarate	HIV-1 infection
5	Vaxelis	Hexavalent vaccine against diphtheria, pertussis, tetanus, poliomyelitis, hepatitis B and *Haemophilus influenzae* type b infections

Appendix 4: Drugs Safety Alerts

	Drug	Safety alerts
1.	Enasidenib Ivosidenib	Signs and symptoms of a life-threatening side effect called differentiation syndrome are not being recognized in patients receiving these drugs.
2.	Alemtuzumab	Serious cases of stroke and tears in the lining of arteries in the head and neck have occurred in patients with multiple sclerosis shortly after treatment with alemtuzumab.
3.	Fingolimod	Severe worsening of multiple sclerosis after stopping fingolimod.
4.	SGLT-2 inhibitors	Fournier's gangrene
5.	Azithromycin	Long-term azithromycin should not be prescribed for prophylaxis of bronchiolitis obliterans syndrome in patients undergoing donor stem cell transplants because of the increased potential for cancer relapse and death.
6.	Fluoroquinolones	• Hypoglycemia, leading to coma can occur in the elderly and diabetics on oral hypoglycemic medications or insulin. • Disturbance in attention, memory impairment, and delirium are new adverse reactions to be added to the labels of the entire class of fluoroquinolones. • Aortic aneurysm • Aortic dissection
7.	Benzocaine	Oral drug products containing benzocaine should not be used to treat infants and children younger than 2 years owing to the risk of methemoglobinemia.
8.	Dolutegravir	Neural tube birth defects
9.	Lamotrigine	Serious immune system reaction called hemophagocytic lymphohistiocytosis (HLH)
10.	Clarithromycin	Caution before prescribing to patients with heart disease because of a potential increased risk of heart problems or death that can occur years later.
11.	Obeticholic acid	Daily dose in patients with moderate to severe primary biliary cholangitis, a rare chronic liver disease, increases the risk of serious liver injury, hence should be administered once weekly.
12.	Loperamide	Limit the number of doses in a package owing to the increased reports of serious heart problems and deaths, with much higher than the recommended doses of loperamide, primarily among people who are intentionally misusing or abusing the product, despite the addition of a warning to the medicine label and a previous communication.

Contd...

13. Opioid cough and cold medicines	Use limited to >18 years of age because the risks of these medicines outweigh their benefits in children younger than 18 years.

Selected References for Further Reading

1. Adams D, Suhr OB, Dyck PJ, Litchy WJ, Leahy RG, Chen J, Gollob J, Coelho T (2017). Trial design and rationale for APOLLO, a Phase 3, placebo-controlled study of patisiran in patients with hereditary ATTR amyloidosis with polyneuropathy. BMC neurology, 17(1), 181. doi:10.1186/s12883-017-0948-5
2. Balestrini S and Sisodiya SM (2016). Audit of use of stiripentol in adults with Dravet syndrome. Acta neurologica Scandinavica, 135(1), 73-79.
3. Blair HA (2018). Duvelisib: First Global Approval. Drugs. doi:10.1007/s40265-018-1013-4
4. Busse P, Farkas H, Banerji A, Lumry W, Longhurst H, Sexton D and Riedl M (2018). Lanadelumab for the Prophylactic Treatment of Hereditary Angioedema with C1 Inhibitor Deficiency: A Review of Preclinical and Phase I Studies. Biodrugs, 33(1), 33-43. doi: 10.1007/s40259-018-0325-y
5. Celio L and Fabbroni C (2018). Pro-netupitant/palonosetron (IV) for the treatment of radio-and-chemotherapy-induced nausea and vomiting. Expert Opinion On Pharmacotherapy, 19(11), 1267-1277. doi: 10.1080/14656566.2018.1494726
6. Colombier M and Molina J (2018). Doravirine/: a review, 13(4), 308-314. https://doi.org/10.1097/COH.0000000000000471
7. Deeks E (2019). Sarecycline: First Global Approval. Drugs. doi: 10.1007/s40265-019-1053-4
8. Detke HC, Goadsby PJ, Wang S, Friedman DI, Selzler KJ and Aurora SK (2018). Galcanezumab in chronic migraine: The randomized, double-blind, placebo-controlled REGAIN study. Neurology, 91(24), e2211-e2221.
9. Devinsky O, Cilio MR, Cross H, Fernandez-Ruiz J, French J, Hill C, Katz R, Di Marzo V, Jutras-Aswad D, Notcutt WG, Martinez-Orgado J, Robson PJ, Rohrback BG, Thiele E, Whalley B, Friedman D (2014). Cannabidiol: pharmacology and potential therapeutic role in epilepsy and other neuropsychiatric disorders. Epilepsia, 55(6), 791-802.
10. Dhillon S (2018). Ivosidenib: First Global Approval. Drugs, 78(14), 1509-1516.
11. Dhillon S (2018). Moxetumomab Pasudotox: First Global Approval. Drugs, 78(16), 1763-1767.
12. Doughty B, Morgenson D and Brooks T (2019). Lofexidine: A Newly FDA-Approved, Nonopioid Treatment for Opioid Withdrawal. Annals of Pharmacotherapy, 106002801982895. doi:10.1177/10600280198 28954

13. Forsythe A, Arondekar B, Tremblay G, Chan G, Su Y (2017) Systematic literature review and indirect treatment comparisons (ITC) of glasdegib (GLAS) plus low dose ara-c (LDAC) versus a hypomethylating agent (HMA) for previously untreated acute myeloid leukemia (AML) patients ineligible for intensive chemotherapy (NIC). doi: 10.1200/jco.2017.35.15_suppl.e18526

14. Iacob S and Iacob D (2017). Ibalizumab Targeting CD4 Receptors, An Emerging Molecule in HIV Therapy. Frontiers In Microbiology, 8. doi: 10.3389/fmicb.2017.02323

15. Insogna KL, Briot K, Imel EA, Kamenický P, Ruppe MD, Portale AA, Carpenter TO; AXLES 1 Investigators. (2018). A Randomized, Double-Blind, Placebo-Controlled, Phase 3 Trial Evaluating the Efficacy of Burosumab, an Anti-FGF23 Antibody, in Adults With X-Linked Hypophosphatemia: Week 24 Primary Analysis. Journal of Bone and Mineral Research, 33(8), 1383-1393. doi:10.1002/jbmr.3475

16. Kaplon H and Reichert J (2018). Antibodies to watch in 2018. Mabs, 10(2), 183-203. doi: 10.1080/19420862.2018.1415671

17. Keam SJ (2018). Inotersen: First Global Approval. Drugs. doi:10.1007/s40265-018-0968-5

18. Kim E (2015). Lusutrombopag: First Global Approval. Drugs, 76(1), 155-158. doi: 10.1007/s40265-015-0525-4

19. Koshkin VS and Small EJ (2018). Apalutamide in the treatment of castrate-resistant prostate cancer: evidence from clinical trials. Therapeutic advances in urology, 10(12), 445-454. doi:10.1177/1756287218811450

20. Kotyla PJ (2018). Are Janus Kinase Inhibitors Superior over Classic Biologic Agents in RA Patients?. BioMed research international, 2018, 7492904. doi:10.1155/2018/7492904

21. Kumar P, Richmond G, Win S, Weinheimer S PhD, Marsolais C, Lewis S (2018). Phase 3 Study of Ibalizumab for Multidrug- Resistant HIV-1, 645-654. https://doi.org/10.1056/NEJMoa1711460

22. Lattanzi S, Brigo F, Trinka E, Vernieri F, Corradetti T, Dobran M and Silvestrini M (2019). Erenumab for Preventive Treatment of Migraine: A Systematic Review and Meta-Analysis of Efficacy and Safety. Drugs. doi:10.1007/s40265-019-01069-1

23. LiZ, Alyamani M, Li J, Rogacki K, Abazeed M, Upadhyay SK, Balk S P., Taplin ME, Auchus RJ, Sharifi N. (2016). Redirecting abiraterone metabolism to fine-tune prostate cancer anti-androgen therapy. Nature, 533(7604), 547-51.

24. Lovejoy C, Meara I, Long P, Hruby DE and PhD. (2018). of Smallpox. https://doi.org/10.1056/NEJMoa1705688

25. Markham A (2018). Ibalizumab: First Global Approval. Drugs, 78(7), 781-785. https://doi.org/10.1007/s40265-018-0907-5

26. McKeage K (2019). Ravulizumab: First Global Approval. Drugs. doi:10.1007/s40265-019-01068-2

27. Meaney CJ, Beccari MV, Yang Y and Zhao J (2017). Systematic Review and Meta-Analysis of Patiromer and Sodium Zirconium Cyclosilicate: A New Armamentarium for the Treatment of Hyperkalemia. Pharmacotherapy, 37(4), 401-411.

28. Newland A, Lee E, McDonald V and Bussel J (2018). Fostamatinib for persistent/chronic adult immune thrombocytopenia. Immunotherapy, 10(1), 9-25. doi: 10.2217/imt-2017-0097

29. Oh S, Shcherbakova N, Kostera-Pruszczyk A, Alsharabati M, Dimachkie M and Blanco J, et al. (2016). Amifampridine phosphate (Firdapse®) is effective and safe in a phase 3 clinical trial in LEMS. Muscle & Nerve, 53(5), 717-725. doi: 10.1002/mus.25070

30. Omoto S, Speranzini V, Hashimoto T, Nosh T, Yamaguchi H, Kawai M, Shishido T (2018). Characterization of influenza virus variants induced by treatment with the endonuclease inhibitor baloxavir marboxil, (April), 1-15. https://doi.org/10.1038/s41598-018-27890-4

31. Perl AE, Altman JK, Cortes J, Smith C, Litzow M, Baer MR, Levis M (2017). Selective inhibition of FLT3 by gilteritinib in relapsed or refractory acute myeloid leukaemia: a multicentre, first-in-human, open-label, phase 1-2 study. The Lancet Oncology, 18(8), 1061-1075. doi:10.1016/s1470-2045(17)30416-3

32. Quinn D, Barnes C, Yates W, Bourdet D, Moran E and Potgieter P, et al (2018). Pharmacodynamics, pharmacokinetics and safety of revefenacin (TD-4208), a long-acting muscarinic antagonist, in patients with chronic obstructive pulmonary disease (COPD): Results of two randomized, double-blind, phase 2 studies. Pulmonary Pharmacology & Therapeutics, 48, 71-79. doi: 10.1016/j.pupt.2017.10.003

33. Sax P, Pozniak A, Montes M, Koenig E, DeJesus E and Stellbrink H, et al (2017). Coformulated bictegravir, emtricitabine, and tenofovir alafenamide versus dolutegravir with emtricitabine and tenofovir alafenamide, for initial treatment of HIV-1 infection (GS-US-380-1490): a randomised, double-blind, multicentre, phase 3, non-inferiority trial. The Lancet, 390(10107), 2073-2082. doi: 10.1016/s0140-6736(17)32340-1

34. Solomkin J, Evans D, Slepavicius A, Lee P, Marsh A and Tsai L, et al (2017). Assessing the Efficacy and Safety of Eravacycline vs Ertapenem in Complicated Intra-abdominal Infections in the Investigating Gram-Negative Infections Treated With Eravacycline (IGNITE 1) Trial. JAMA Surgery, 152(3), 224. doi: 10.1001/jamasurg.2016.4237

35. Sun J, Zager JS and Eroglu Z (2018). Encorafenib/binimetinib for the treatment of BRAF-mutant advanced, unresectable, or metastatic melanoma: design, development, and potential place in therapy. OncoTargets and therapy, 11, 9081-9089. doi:10.2147/OTT.S171693

36. Taylor HS, Giudice LC, Lessey BA, Abrao MS, Kotarski J, Archer DF, Chwalisz K (2017). Treatment of Endometriosis-Associated Pain with Elagolix, an Oral GnRH Antagonist. New England Journal of Medicine, 377(1), 28-40. doi:10.1056/nejmoa1700089

37. Thomas J, Levy H, Amato S, Vockley J, Zori R, Dimmock D, Northrup H (2018). Pegvaliase for the treatment of phenylketonuria: Results of a long-term phase 3 clinical trial program (PRISM). Molecular Genetics and Metabolism, 124(1), 27-38. doi:10.1016/j.ymgme.2018.03.006

38. VanderPluym J, Dodick DW, Lipton RB, Ma Y, Loupe PS and Bigal ME (2018). Fremanezumab for preventive treatment of migraine: Functional status on headache-free days. Neurology, 91(12), e1152-e1165.

39. Villano S, Steenbergen J and Loh E (2016). Omadacycline: development of a novel aminomethylcycline antibiotic for treating drug-resistant bacterial infections. Future Microbiology, 11(11), 1421-1434. doi: 10.2217/fmb-2016-0100

40. Warnock DG, Bichet DG, Holida M, Goker-Alpan O, Nicholls K, Thomas M, Eyskens F, Johnson FK (2015). Oral Migalastat HCl Leads to Greater Systemic Exposure and Tissue Levels of Active α-Galactosidase A in Fabry Patients when Co-Administered with Infused Agalsidase. PloS one, 10(8), e0134341. doi:10.1371/journal.pone.0134341

41. Woodfield SE, Zhang L, Scorsone KA, Liu Y and Zage PE (2016). Binimetinib inhibits MEK and is effective against neuroblastoma tumor cells with low NF1 expression. BMC cancer, 16, 172. doi:10.1186/s12885-016-2199-z